THE ESSENTIAL

Guide to Medical Staff Reappointment

Beverly E. Pybus, CMSC

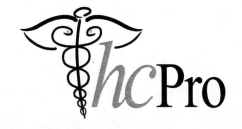

Beverly E. Pybus, CMSC, Author
Rena Cutchin, Senior Managing Editor
Erin Ellis, Managing Editor
Jean St. Pierre, Creative Director
Mike Mirabello, Senior Graphic Artist
Matthew Sharpe, Graphic Artist
Steve DeGrappo, Cover Designer
Crystal Blodgett, Layout Artist
Dale Seamans, Executive Editor
Suzanne Perney, Publisher

Advice given is general. Readers should consult professional counsel for specific legal, ethical, or clinical questions.

Arrangements can be made for quantity discounts.

For more information, contact:

HCPro
P.O. Box 1168
Marblehead, MA 01945
Telephone: 800/650-6787 or 781/639-1872
Fax: 781/639-2982
E-mail: *customerservice@hcpro.com*

Visit HCPro at its World Wide Web sites:
www.hcmarketplace.com, www.hcpro.com, and www.himinfo.com.

11/2003
18348

Contents

List of figures

About the Author

Beverly E. Pybus, CMSC

Beverly E. Pybus, CMSC, is senior consultant for credentialing and privileging services for The Greeley Company, a division of HCPro, Inc, in Marblehead, MA. Prior to joining The Greeley Company, Pybus was principal of The Beverly Group, a health care consulting firm based in Georgetown, MA. As principal of The Beverly Group, she was responsible for the management and direction of consulting projects in medical staff and allied health professional credentialing, and customized clinical privileging systems.

She has worked with medical staff and health care organizations across the country to design practical, up-to-date credentialing and core privileging systems and to help resolve the sensitive issues that often accompany credentialing decisions.

Pybus was a senior health care consultant for eight years with InterQual, Inc., where she was a member of the faculty for its educational programs, as well as a contributor to the development of credentialing software and numerous publications.

Pybus has specialized in corporate management strategies with previous experience in legal, private, and educational organizations as well as health-related facilities. Beverly is the author and editor of numerous articles and books about credentialing and privileging, including *A Guide to Centralized Credentialing: Evaluating Current Issues and Trends* and *Privileging Quick Reference Guide, Second Edition.* She is co-author of *Core Privileges: A Practical Approach to Development and Implementation* and *A Guide to AHP Credentialing: Challenges and Opportunities to Credentialing Allied Health Professionals*, all published by HCPro, Inc.

Pybus holds a certificate in risk management, a certificate in mediation, and is certified by the National Association Medical Staff Services. Pybus is a member of the American Health Lawyers Association's Credentialing and Peer Review Practice Group.

Chapter 1

Credentialing:

The prerequisite

to reappointment

CHAPTER 1

Credentialing: The prerequisite to reappointment

Competent health care practitioners form the foundation of quality patient care. But in today's complex health care environment, no practitioner is competent to provide every service and treatment, and a few are not competent to provide any patient care. With continuously mounting legal and regulatory pressures, as well as ever-increasing media coverage of health care quality issues, all health care organizations are under more scrutiny now than ever to make sure those who provide patient care are competent to do so.

To ensure that only qualified, competent practitioners provide patient care, health care organizations thoroughly review each applicant's qualifications at both initial appointment and reappointment. Reappointment is a crucial component of a health care organization's quality and performance improvement efforts; it gives the organization the opportunity to regularly reevaluate each medical staff member's clinical skills, competency, and professional conduct. It also provides the opportunity to determine whether an individual still meets the organization's expectations, requirements, and membership and privileging criteria.

The process of collecting, reviewing, and assessing physicians' qualifications to make such determinations is commonly referred to as credentialing. Credentialing is the prerequisite to reappointment. After all, if organizations don't collect adequate information at initial appointment, the basis for a thorough reevaluation will be weak.

Reasons to credential

One of the more straightforward reasons why hospitals credential their physicians is because the Joint Commission on Accreditation of Healthcare Organizations (JCAHO) requires it. Specifically, the intent statement of the JCAHO's 2003 Medical Staff standards **MS.5–MS.5.1.3** and the over-view section of the 2004 Medical Staff chapter state that hospitals must, at minimum, credential all licensed independent practitioners (LIPs), or practitioners permitted by law to provide patient care without direct supervision.

Although the types of practitioners recognized as LIPs vary from state to state, all states regard physicians, dentists, and podiatrists as LIPs. Some states also consider psychologists as part of the LIP family.

Note: As this book went to press, the JCAHO had introduced its latest round of standards revisions, scheduled to take effect on January 1, 2004. For the purposes of this book, any reference made to a particular Medical Staff standard will list the 2003 standard as well as the 2004 standard.

Upon medical staff appointment, physicians must apply for clinical privileges (i.e., permission to perform specific procedures or to treat specific conditions). Some hospitals also allow certain non-physician practitioners to apply for clinical privileges. The process that hospitals follow to grant clinical privileges is often called "privileges delineation," or privileging. See Chapter 4 for a more detailed discussion of privileging and its role in the reappointment process.

The prospect of creating effective, efficient credentialing and privileging systems intimidates many hospitals. While the ultimate goal of every credentialing and privileging system should be to ensure quality patient care, hospitals also must consider the following additional factors:

- Compliance with federal and state regulations such as the Americans With Disabilities Act (ADA)[1]
- Compliance with regulatory and accrediting agencies such as the Centers for Medicare & Medicaid Services, JCAHO, National Committee for Quality Assurance (NCQA), American Accreditation Association for Ambulatory Health Care, and other applicable accrediting agencies
- Elimination of internal medical staff conflicts and "turf battles"
- Minimization of legal risk
- Attraction of health care purchasers
- Enhancement of overall organization marketability

The credentialing process

The credentialing process involves the following four main steps:

---

[1] The ADA (42 U.S.C. 1211[a]) prohibits a health care facility from denying or restricting a practitioner's clinical privileges based on a health condition or a perceived disability, unless the health condition prevents the practitioner from exercising the privilege safely in the care of patients, and unless there is no reasonable accommodations the health care entity can make to enable the practitioner to exercise the privilege safely.

1. Create good policies and procedures

In this first step, hospitals create the policies and procedures that define the credentialing process. Hospitals and their medical staffs incorporate into these policies the criteria they will use to make decisions regarding medical staff appointment and clinical privileges delineation. These criteria enable hospitals to eliminate applications that would inevitably face denial if allowed to proceed through the complete credentialing process. To avoid unnecessary denials and the subsequent responsibility of reporting those denials to the National Practitioner Data Bank (NPDB), every hospital should include in its policies minimum criteria that each medical staff applicant must meet before the organization will process his or her application.

In addition to making the credentialing and privileging process more efficient, determining these criteria in advance also makes it more objective. As a result, using criteria reduces the likelihood of a fair hearing when an application is denied. Hospitals should communicate these criteria to all potential applicants, instructing them to apply only if they meet the minimum criteria. (Chapter 6 addresses fair hearings and benchmarking surveys in more detail. Chapter 4 discusses the various methods used to develop a privileging system, including the development of threshold criteria.)

2. Gather information

During this second step, medical staff office personnel review the application and make sure it is complete. Then they conduct primary-source verification, which is crucial in determining the authenticity of the information provided by the applicant. Medical staff office personnel verify each piece of information on the application with its primary source, or the issuer of the credential (e.g., the medical school that issued the MD or DO degree). The medical staff office should clarify with the applicant any discrepancies between the information on the application and the information obtained from primary sources before moving it to the next stage. No application should take the next step until it is complete and the hospital receives all the information it needs to properly evaluate the applicant's qualifications.

3. Evaluate and recommend

During this stage, the appropriate department chair(s), the credentials committee, and the medical executive committee evaluate the application and its supporting documentation. This evaluation should focus on whether the information in the completed application adequately demonstrates that the applicant meets the criteria for membership and privileges, as established in the policies and procedures.

4. Review and grant

During this step, the hospital's governing board reviews all recommendations concerning the application and makes a final decision to grant or deny medical staff membership/privileges.

The rules of credentialing

As stated earlier, the ultimate goal of credentialing is to ensure quality patient care. A hospital's credentialing policies and procedures should reflect that goal. Therefore, when developing credentialing policies and procedures, hospitals should keep the following rules in mind:

1. Place the burden on the applicant

Some hospitals feel compelled to expend significant amounts of administrative and staff time verifying the qualifications of practitioners who apply for medical staff appointment with or without clinical privileges. Every hospital should make clear in its policies and in practice that the applicant is responsible for providing the hospital with the information it needs to make an informed decision and to resolve any doubts regarding appointment and/or clinical privileges. A hospital should not waste valuable time and labor trying to verify information on an application or reapplication or coaxing reluctant references to respond.

2. Establish clear and rigorous appointment and clinical privileges criteria for applicants

The hospital should never be forced to deny medical staff appointment because of an applicant's or reapplicant's inadequate education, training, and experience; these are shortcomings that a hospital can easily identify when it receives the application or reapplication from the practitioner. A good credentialing process should start with threshold criteria and objective preapplication screening. If a hospital considers a practitioner who lacks specific, defined training or fails to meet education re-quirements, hospital leaders and staff will waste time and energy processing an application or reapplication that the hospital will inevitably deny because the practitioner does not meet qualifications. In addition, a practitioner who is denied appointment and/or privileges might be entitled to a fair hearing—a time-consuming and very costly process. And in most cases, the hospital must report a denial to the NPDB. A sample policy on the responsibility for NPDB querying and reporting appears in Appendix D on p. 253. See Figure 1.1 on p. 11 for sample policy and procedure for placing the burden on the applicant.

3. Continuously improve credentialing practices and procedures

Hospitals are sometimes reluctant to upgrade credentialing policies and procedures, arguing that it is not fair to require new applicants to meet more rigorous requirements than existing members. This is simply the wrong attitude. The practice of medicine—and therefore the medical education and clinical experience of applicants—is constantly changing. As a result, the criteria for clinical privileges must reflect those changes. Sound, rigorous standards should never need justification. Chapter 2 contains recommendations for evaluating your credentialing process on an annual basis. (See p. 15.)

4. Do not confuse appointment to the medical staff with the granting of clinical privileges

Too often, medical staffs, hospital managers, and governing board members confuse medical staff appointment with the granting of clinical privileges. Medical staff appointment simply permits an individual to participate in the medical staff organization. Clinical privileges, on the other hand, specify the particular clinical activities an individual may exercise in the hospital based on his or her education, training, and experience. An individual can be appointed to the medical staff but have no clinical privileges. Likewise, an individual can hold clinical privileges without being appointed to the medical staff. (Chapter 4 addresses the various approaches and aspects of clinical privileging, and Chapter 7 discusses practitioners with few or no clinical privileges who could be members of the medical staff.)

5. Collect clinical data and references

In the past, hospitals have not routinely requested information about the numbers and types of procedures that a practitioner has performed. Without sufficient clinical information that shows the applicant is clinically competent to perform the requested procedures or treatments, hospitals should consider that privilege request incomplete and cease to process it. Hospitals should require that every request for clinical privileges include data regarding the number and types of clinical activities the practitioner has performed, as well as the time period(s) in which he or she performed them. This data is especially important at reappointment when some practitioners may have a very low volume of activity at the hospital. Chapter 7 discusses the problems associated with low-volume practitioners and offers possible solutions.

6. Send only complete applications to department chairs/credentials committee for review

Administrative personnel sometimes feel it is necessary to send an application or reapplication to department chairs or the credentials committee even though it is incomplete. This may mean either that the hospital has not received certain references or information pertaining to past clinical activity or malpractice cases, or that the hospital has not verified all of the practitioner's credentials. Likewise, some committees make a recommendation for appointment/reappointment even if the practitioner's file does not contain sufficient information. In today's medical and legal environments, it is best to have hospital administration assume nearly all responsibility for assembling the credentials file in compliance with hospital policies and procedures before designated individuals and committees review it. Using a checklist that outlines the documents/information required to complete the file often proves helpful for administrative personnel. (Chapter 3, which covers the reappointment process, contains examples of this type of document.)

7. Use all available resources

Today, hospitals face increasingly complex credentialing issues—such as new medical techniques and procedures—and privilege requests from nonphysician practitioners. When faced with such challenges, hospitals should use all internal resources, or external consultants when it needs specific expertise. (Chapter 5 discusses external peer review—i.e., turning to outside sources for peer review assistance.) Hospitals should also use all available technology—e.g., computer software, the Internet, fax machines, e-mail, etc.) to gather the necessary information to make an informed decision.

8. Be businesslike and professional

Too often, credentialing professionals assume that nearly all practitioners are courteous, professional, caring, and collegial. Although many practitioners do indeed possess these qualities, it is important to realize that credentialing activities occasionally result in hurt feelings, anger, hostility, and in some cases, lawsuits. Hospital personnel should always follow procedures. Moreover, they should document that they have done so. Finally, they should make sure the language in all letters and other forms of communication is courteous and businesslike.

The 'evolving credentialing standard'

Currently, JCAHO and NCQA standards provide an excellent starting point for conducting credentialing activities in hospitals and other health care organizations. However, physician leaders and credentialing professionals who take credentialing and privileging very seriously are now discussing an "evolving credentialing standard," which includes steps that go beyond the minimum credentialing standards currently required by the JCAHO, NCQA, and licensing authorities. Recent events have proven that hospitals and other organizations place themselves and their patients at risk if they only follow minimum requirements. One of the more notable events is the September 2000 conviction of Michael Swango, the ex-physician now serving a life prison sentence for murdering three of his patients at a Long Island, NY, hospital in 1993. He is believed to have fatally poisoned seven patients while practicing in a rural village in Zimbabwe from November 1994 to July 1995. A quick background check would have uncovered abruptly curtailed residency programs and a criminal conviction in Swango's past—two obvious warning signs that would have prevented hospitals from appointing him to their medical staffs.

Incidents such as this show why it is necessary for credentialing professionals and medical staff/ hospital leaders to be governed by solid credentialing policies that prohibit recommendations concerning a practitioner's employment, appointment, or clinical privileges until all of the following information has been obtained, verified, and documented, complete with dates, locations, and other relevant facts, such as:

- Lifetime licensure history, including licenses currently or previously held in any allied health discipline
- Lifetime medical education and training history, including all professional schools attended and all approved or non-approved residency programs attended
- Previous 10-year malpractice history, including all claims and settlements

- Specialty board status, including admissibility and board exams taken, passed, or failed
- Sanctions, including those imposed by any organization having a responsibility for overseeing the quality, appropriateness, ethics, or other professional conduct of the practitioner
- Lifetime criminal record (where permitted by law), including all relevant details of the charge and final deposition
- Health care–related employment and appointment history, including terminations, pending challenges/decisions, voluntary resignations/relinquishments, and pending investigations
- Signed professional references (concerning adequacy of clinical knowledge, technical skill, judgment, ability to relate to others, overall professional performance, adherence to rules and bylaws, and health status) by knowledgeable practitioners who have observed the applicant first-hand
- In addition to the above eight elements, hospitals should also consider each applicant's past 12 months of clinical activity (approximate number, type, and location of patients treated)
- Review for consistency between applicant information and information obtained from other sources

The evolving credentialing standard was developed out of the recognition that mistakes in credentialing are attributable to two types of failures. The first is mechanical failure. Mechanical failure means the hospital's failure or inability to collect all relevant information concerning a new applicant for appointment or clinical privileges. Mechanical failure occasionally results from the absence of policies and procedures that require the collection of all appropriate information. Under other circumstances, mechanical failure is due to an organization's inability to obtain information even when it believes such information is necessary for decision-making.

The second type is decision failure. Decision failure occurs when those entrusted with appointment/privileging recommendations approve an applicant even though his or her competence/background is questionable. Chapter 10 provides more detailed information about these and other issues.

The evolving credentialing standard is intended to assist organizations in eliminating the possibility of mechanical failure. In the presence of all of the information outlined above, it would be difficult for a decision-maker to inadvertently make a mistake concerning appointment or the granting of clinical privileges.

The standard also represents a fairly logical evolution of credentialing procedures that recognizes the complexities of today's medical field. Physicians change positions far more frequently today. Unfortunately, some do so to hide a history of poor care, disciplinary actions, and even criminal conviction.

Note: The evolving credentialing standard is not an actual required standard set forth by the JCAHO, NCQA, or any other accrediting body. However, it is highly recommended that organizations adopt it as a sound approach to thorough, high-quality credentialing. To ensure patient safety and safeguard against liability, health care organizations must go above and beyond the customarily acceptable approaches.

Hospitals should review the evolving credentialing standard and consider adopting it. If they choose to adopt the standard, they should modify it and continue to treat credentialing as the professional and patient-focused activity that it has become. After all, the relatively minor cost of checking physicians' qualifications is easily justified by patients' faith and trust in their health care organizations.

Figure 1.1

Sample policy and procedure: Placing the burden on the applicant

Policy

Each individual practitioner who applies for or maintains medical staff membership/privileges has the burden of providing evidence that demonstrates, under the sole discretion of the hospital, that he or she meets the hospital's established criteria for membership and privileges. This policy applies at the time of initial appointment, reappointment, clinical privileges request, employment, or any time during a practitioner's affiliation with the institution.

Procedure

To fulfill this responsibility, the practitioner has the burden of producing any information requested by the hospital or its authorized representatives that is reasonably necessary, under the sole discretion of the hospital, to evaluate whether he or she meets the established criteria for medical staff membership and privileges.

If there is undue delay in obtaining such required information, or if the hospital requires clarification of such information, the medical staff office will request the applicant's assistance. Under these circumstances, the medical staff may modify its usual and customary time periods for processing the application or reapplication. The hospital has sole discretion for determining what is an adequate response.

If during the process of initial application or reapplication the applicant fails to respond adequately within 30 days to a request for further information or assistance, the hospital will deem the application or reapplication as voluntarily withdrawn. The result of the withdrawal is automatic termination of the application or reapplication process. The hospital will not consider the termination an adverse action. Therefore, the applicant or reapplicant is not entitled to a fair hearing or appeal consistent with the medical staff's fair hearing plan. The hospital will not report the action to any external agency (e.g., medical licensing board or NPDB).

Chapter 2

Credentials Files:

Content,

maintenance,

access, and

confidentiality

Credentials Files: Content, maintenance, access, and confidentiality

Complete, organized, and updated credentialing files are essential to the reappointment process. Your credentials files are the central repository for all information regarding a practitioner's clinical privileges, quality of care, and medical staff membership status. Well-organized credentials files ensure compliance with Joint Commission on Accreditation of Healthcare Organizations standards and ensure that the hospital's decisions concerning a practitioner's application for reappointment and clinical privileges are based on reliable information.

Note: See the end of this chapter for policies about content, access, control, retention, and confidentiality of practitioner credentials files and information.

Maintenance and storage concerns

The issue of appropriate storage mechanisms is largely administrative, and management has the authority to determine the format in which such files will be stored. Most credentials files contain large amounts of material that is extraneous to the credentials function (e.g., letters received thanking physicians for service on committees, copies of old continuing medical education files, etc.). Purge credentials files to considerably reduce the overall volume. An institution interested in minimizing the number of documents within each credentials file should first establish a policy that indicates what must be maintained and what information can be eliminated from the file without compromising the institution's future ability to defend itself in a corporate negligence case or provide information to other facilities.

Tip: Consider storing credentials files in a scanned, digitized, or any other electronic form. This typically saves space.

Note: Maintain the credentialing files of practitioners who no longer provide care at your facility for a period of seven to 21 years. If the practitioner ever treated an infant or pediatric patient, it is widely recommended that the file be maintained for at least 21 years. If the practitioner treated only adults it would likely be acceptable to maintain the file for only seven years. Because individual state laws and regulations vary on this issue, seek advice from an experienced health care attorney regarding the issue of "age of retention."

Figure 2.1 — Elements of a credentials file

The following documents—as applicable to the particular facility—should be included in a complete practitioner credentials file. This document can also be used as a checklist for updating and ensuring that the file is complete.

Initial appointment: Application

❑ Applicant's letter requesting appointment to the medical staff with clinical privileges
❑ Typed, completed, and signed application form
❑ Completed request for clinical privileges form
❑ Practitioner's release of liability statement
❑ Three letters of recommendation sent directly to the chief executive officer from persons who have recently worked with the applicant, directly observed his or her professional performance over a reasonable period of time, and who will provide reliable information regarding the practitioner's current clinical ability, ethical character, and ability to work with others. References must be from individuals practicing in a field similar to the applicant.

Note: These references are optional.

Initial appointment: Information gathering

❑ At least three questionnaires attesting to judgment, skill, professional performance, and clinical knowledge from individuals identified in the credentials policy manual
❑ Letter to applicant requesting additional information to complete application (if any)
❑ Response to above request
❑ Letter to applicant regarding processing of application (if any)
❑ Initial application processing checklist (if used)
❑ Verification of professional liability insurance and claims experience
❑ Information from all prior and current insurance carriers concerning claims, suits, and settlements (if any) during the past 10 years
❑ Letter accompanying clinical reference questionnaire (if used)
❑ Clinical reference questionnaire(s),
❑ Letter accompanying administrative questionnaire (if any)
❑ Verification and copy of certificates and documentation from an appropriate specialty board attesting to board status

Figure 2.1 — Elements of a credentials file (cont.)

❏ Letter requesting verification of license

❏ Verification of licensure status in all current or past states of licensure

❏ Letter to Federation of State Medical Boards (FSMB) requesting verification of all licenses (if used)

❏ FSMB report

❏ AMA Physician Masterfile Profile—or its equivalent (if used)

❏ National Practitioner Data Bank report

❏ Letter and response requesting additional information from applicant (if any)

❏ Telephone contact report(s)

❏ Interview report(s) (if used)

Initial appointment: Review and action

❏ Department chair's report and recommendation

❏ Credentials committee's review and recommendation/report

❏ Request for temporary privileges (if any)

❏ Letter to applicant regarding deferral of appointment request

❏ Letter to applicant regarding denial or modification of appointment request

❏ Letter to applicant regarding approval of medical staff appointment

❏ A signed agreement that the individual was oriented to the medical staff bylaws, policies, and procedures, and that he or she agrees to follow them when admitting patients and providing patient care (if used)

❏ Applicant-specific provisional status guidelines

❏ Letter to appointee regarding proctoring procedures, if applicable

❏ Proctor's report(s) (if any)

❏ Letter accompanying provisional status report

❏ Provisional status report and department chair recommendations to conclude provisional period

❏ Letter to department chair regarding extension of provisional period

❏ Letter from department chair regarding extension of provisional period

Initial appointment: Application

❏ Letter/notice to appointee regarding reappointment

Figure 2.1   Elements of a credentials file (cont.)

❑ Completed reappointment request and information form
❑ Completed request for clinical privileges
❑ Current clinical privilege forms and clinical activity
❑ Request for modification of clinical privileges
❑ Practitioner's release of liability statement

Reappointment: Information gathering
❑ Monitoring form (if used)
❑ Letter requesting information from other practice settings
❑ Questionnaires pertaining to reappointment of physician
❑ Letter to appointee requesting assistance in obtaining information for reappointment application (if any)
❑ Reappointment activity summary
❑ Request for an investigation/corrective action
❑ Verification (copy of certificates or a copy of a letter from an appropriate specialty board) of board status (i.e., board admissibility or board certification)
❑ Department chair's report on privileges request form
❑ Evidence of continuing medical education
❑ Attendance record for required medical staff and department meetings (if required)
❑ Record of service on medical staff, department, and hospital committees
❑ Quality assurance/utilization review monitoring reports
❑ Evidence of current license
❑ Evidence of current malpractice insurance

Other
❑ Incident reports
❑ Certifications (e.g., DEA, ACLS)
❑ Reports of any investigations and/or disciplinary action
❑ Data bank reports (e.g., NPDB, FSMB, AMA)
❑ Specific experience and successful results that form the basis for granting requested privileges and reappointment

Figure 2.1   Elements of a credentials file (cont.)

❑ Practitioner profile report on membership, citizenship, clinical activity

❑ Leave of absence request/reinstatement

❑ Military leave of absence request/reinstatement

Reappointment: Review and action

❑ Department chair's report and recommendation on membership and clinical privileges

❑ Credentials committee's review and recommendation

❑ Medical executive committee's review and recommendation

❑ Request for temporary privileges (if any)

❑ Letter to applicant—Deferral of reappointment request

❑ Letter to applicant—Denial or modification of reappointment request

❑ Letter to Applicant—Approval of medical staff reappointment and clinical privileges

❑ Evidence of governing board review and action

Note: Incident reports, patient complaints, quality review data are generally kept separately from the practitioner credentials file in either the quality improvement department or the medical staff office.

| Figure 2.2 | Credentials file: Content, access, control, and retention policy |

Policy

A credentials file shall be maintained for each applicant for medical staff membership and/or affiliation as an allied health professional. These files are confidential and shall be secured in the medical staff services department under the direct control of the director of medical staff services. Access shall be limited to those individuals and released in the manner set forth in the policy entitled, "Confidentiality of Medical Staff Information and Policies." (Note: See Figure 2.3 for that policy.)

File content

The credentials file must include the components outlined below.

Correspondence includes the following:

- Correspondence to and from the applicant related to the preapplication, application, verification, and review/approval processes.
- Correspondence related directly to the applicant's citizenship as a member/affiliate (i.e., committee appointments/removals, notification of medical record suspension).
- Correspondence to the practitioner related to clinical performance. Letters of complaint or incident reports to the practitioner are not automatically filed in the practitioner's file. They are handled in accordance with hospital policy and referred through appropriate channels. However, if such items result in correspondence to the practitioner/corrective action, the resultant correspondence/notification to the practitioner shall become a permanent part of the file.

Note: Attorney and client correspondence (e.g., correspondence from the corporate legal office to the hospital regarding a practitioner) SHALL NOT be included in the practitioner's credentials file. Memos from the corporate legal office regarding documentation for a file shall be filed when the memo indicates same.

Demographics include the following:

- Profiles from database
- Original application
- Curriculum vitae
- Consent forms

Figure 2.2	**Credentials file: Content, access, control, and retention policy (cont.)**

Reappointment/Reappraisal includes the following:

- Correspondence related to the reappointment verification and review/approval processes
- Profiles of performance from the process of monitoring the delivery of patient care and professional conduct

Clinical privileges include the following:

- Application for clinical privileges and any correspondence and supporting documentation to the delineation of privileges request, verification, and review/approval processes

Certificates include the following:

- Certificates of professional liability insurance, federal controlled substance registration, state licensure, and pertinent certificates of continuing medical education and professional certification

Verification process—Initial applicants include the following:

- Documentation related to the verification of an initial applicant's credentials shall include the request and response for each element of the verification process as well as unsolicited letters of reference and the executive summary and tracking forms

Corrective action includes the following:

- Documentation of corrective action taken by the hospital
- Documentation of any disciplinary action taken by outside agencies or other hospitals

Control

- Files shall be controlled by an outguide and logging system. When a practitioner's file is removed from the file cabinet, an outguide shall be inserted indicating the date, time, person removing it, as well as the reason and current placement. When a file is viewed or removed for purposes other than medical staff services personnel or those involved in the professional review and approval process, it shall be logged with the date, time, and person reviewing, as well as the reason for removal.

Figure 2.2

Credentials file: Content, access, control, and retention policy (cont.)

Retention

- Credentials files shall be permanently retained. However, some items within the file shall be purged. See section below on "Purge of information in credentials file."
- Active files shall be maintained in the medical staff services department. Inactive files shall be retained in the medical staff services department for two years past the date the file becomes inactive. These files shall then be archived in accordance with the hospital's procedures for the archival of documents.

Item	Retention
Copies of certificates	
License	Current only
State controlled-substance registration	Current only
Federal controlled-substance registration	Permanent
Professional liability insurance	Current only
Professional certificates	Permanent
External CME (mot supporting clinical privilege requests)	Until logged/summarized
Work papers	
Tracking forms	Until final action by board
Memos/correspondence to facilitate the verification process	Until final action by board
Governance summary form	Until conclusion of provisional period
Verification process	
Cover letters to request verification	Upon response
If no response	Permanent with note indicating reason
Query to and response from NPDB	Permanent
Lists from state licensing board providing verification of licensure, and state controlled substance registration	10 years
Related information which supports the initial application, conclusion or provisional period, interim request for changes in privileges and/or status, reappraisal/ reappointment, and temporary privileges	Permanent

Figure 2.2 — **Credentials file: Content, access, control, and retention policy (cont.)**

Item	Retention
Requests for reference from other hospitals	
Letter/release form/response	Permanent
Correspondence to/from applicant/member/affiliate	
Memos/letter to notify individual of information required	Upon receipt of information
If information not received, follow-up and results of adverse action	Permanent
Requests from practitioner	Permanent
Formal notification regarding appointments/ clinical privileges	Hospital decides
Formal notifications of administrative issues related to an appointment (e.g., committee appointments, medical record suspensions)	Permanent
Addendum to the credentials file by the practitioner	Permanent
Miscellaneous items	
Privilege forms	Permanent
Reappointment summary forms	Permanent
Consent forms	Permanent
Alternate coverage forms	Current only

| Figure 2.3 | Confidentiality of medical staff information and policies |

Policy

The hospital recognizes the need to maintain the confidentiality of all information and activities related to the review of care within the institution to protect the integrity of the review process and the rights of the patients and practitioners. Therefore, strict procedures shall be followed for the conduct of the activities and the collection, maintenance, and access of all information.

Recognizing the importance of preserving the confidentiality of this information, all parties, hospital personnel, members of the medical staff and governing body will respect the confidentiality of all information obtained in connection with their responsibilities. This requirement of confidentiality extends not only to the information documented, but also to discussions and deliberations that take place in conducting the activities.

Definitions

Information includes records of meeting, proceedings and interviews, reports, memoranda, statements, recommendations, findings, evaluations, opinions, conclusions, actions, dates, credentials files, and communications (oral or written) pertaining to activities.

Activities include the credentials process including the application, verification and review processes for membership or clinical privileges, corrective action, and hearing and appellate reviews.

"President" of the hospital shall mean the president or his or her designee.

Maintenance and security precautions

Internal

The official minutes and records of all medical staff committees, ad hoc committees, and credentials files shall be maintained in the medical staff services department under the custody of the director, medical staff services. The files shall be locked, except during those times that the director or an authorized representative is present and able to monitor access in accordance with this policy.

Figure 2.3

Confidentiality of medical staff information and policies (cont.)

Access shall be strictly controlled in accordance with the rules set forth in this policy and procedure.

- Limitations shall be placed on access, input, retrieval and reports through the use of passwords
- Files shall be backed up on a daily basis to magnetic disk or tape

Access

Means of access

All requests for information by persons within the hospital shall be presented to the department director. A record of all requests made and granted shall be maintained. Those requests that require notice to, or approval by, other officials shall be forwarded to those persons by the director.

By persons performing official hospital or medical staff functions

Access to information contained in medical staff records to the extent necessary to perform official functions shall be permitted to the following people:

- Officers of the medical staff
- Applicable clinical department chairs and section heads
- Medical staff committee members
- Members of the governing body
- Medical staff services department personnel
- Hospital legal counsel
- The president of the hospital or designee

By practitioner

A practitioner may view his or her file in the medical staff services department in the presence of department personnel. The practitioner may not remove the file or any part of the file. If the practitioner disagrees with the inclusion of an item in his file, he or she may submit an addendum to the applicable department chair.

Copies of the following pieces of information will be provided upon request:

| Figure 2.3 | **Confidentiality of medical staff information and policies (cont.)** |

- Information from the practitioner
- Correspondence to the practitioner
- Administrative or clinical profiles developed by the hospital
- Certificates
- Clinical privilege forms
- Applications

Any other information that is not noted above must be requested in writing. Such requests will be reviewed by the department director and may require consultation with and approval from hospital legal counsel.

By persons or organizations outside of the hospital

Requests from other health care entities related to the credentials process
All requests shall be in writing on letterhead, indicate the reason for the request, and include a release statement that specifically releases the hospital from liability. It must also be signed by the practitioner within 12 months of the request.

Practitioners with no adverse information on file:
The director of the medical staff services department, credentials committee chair, or department chair may provide information to verify the practitioner's term of affiliation, staff status, and clinical privileges with the hospital. Any other information shall only be provided when specifically requested and only when such information is supported by documentation in the file.

Practitioners with adverse information on file:
The request shall be referred to the respective department chair/president of the staff/president of the hospital for response. It is recommended that consultation from legal counsel be obtained.

Other requests

All other requests for information contained in the medical staff records by persons or organizations

Figure 2.3 | **Confidentiality of medical staff information and policies (cont.)**

outside of the hospital shall be in writing and forwarded to the president of the hospital. The medical executive committee and the governing body may enact release of information policies applying to specific types of requests (e.g., professional review organizations, accreditation bodies, boards of medical examiners, etc.). When such policies release information mandated by state or federal statutes are enacted, they shall be attached to this policy and procedure and shall be controlling.

Subpoenas

All subpoenas of medical staff records shall be referred to hospital legal counsel through the president of the hospital.

Telephone requests

The release of practitioner information requested by telephone shall be limited to confirmation or acknowledgment of a specific practitioner's period of affiliation, staff category, and department/section membership, and information released through the physician referral program.

Chapter 3

The

Reappointment

Process

The Reappointment Process

As stated in Chapter 1, reappointment is a crucial element of a health care organization's quality and performance improvement plan, as it allows the organization to regularly reevaluate each medical staff member's clinical skills and competency to determine whether he or she continues to practice in accordance with the facility's membership and privileging criteria. Ensuring that only excellent, fully qualified, and competent physicians serve on the medical staff not only leads to high-quality care and fosters good will in the community, but it also safeguards the organization from potential litigation. Today, more patients are filing corporate negligence suits against hospitals for poor outcomes caused by physician errors. This trend indicates that, more than ever before, hospitals are being held liable for the actions of their medical staff members.

Hospitals, therefore, should not regard reappointment as simply another Joint Commission on Ac-creditation of Healthcare Organizations (JCAHO) requirement. The creation and implementation of solid, effective policies and procedures are the keys to excellent patient care reduced liability risk.

Where the JCAHO stands

The JCAHO requires in its *Comprehensive Accreditation Manual for Hospitals* that reappointment to the medical staff and the granting, renewal, or revision of clinical privileges must be made for a period of no more than two years (**MS.5.11** in the 2003 version; **MS.4.20** in the 2004 version). Standard **MS.5.12** (**MS.4.20** in 2004 version) also say reappraisal for reappointment to the medical staff or renewal or revision of clinical privileges must be based on ongoing monitoring of

- professional performance
- professional judgment
- clinical or technical skills

Although not required by the JCAHO, hospitals may also choose to look at a practitioner's health status and hospital citizenship status as further reappraisal criteria.

Note: When considering health status at reappointment, organizations must remember to comply with the Americans with Disabilities Act (ADA).

The Americans with Disabilities Act

In an August 1998 decision in Menkowitz v. Pottstown Memorial Hospital Medical Center, the United States Court of Appeals for the Third Circuit decided that a physician member of a hospital medical staff could sue the hospital for alleged discrimination under Title III of the ADA. Until this significant decision, Title III of the ADA had been applied only to hospital employees, not to physicians who held privileges in the hospital, but were not hospital employees. This decision may or may not affect your hospital, but to avoid a potential discrimination lawsuit brought by a physician, take extra care to document evidence that your hospital considered a physician's disability and its effect on patient care and the institutional management only after your hospital reached a decision regarding qualifications for appointment or reappointment. Your hospital should also be able to demonstrate that it carefully considered the effect of the disability on quality of care and that it considered its ability to make reasonable accommodations to prevent the disability from negatively affecting patient care and safety in the hospital.

The reappointment process (see Figure 3.1 on p. 44 for a reappointment flowchart and Figure 3.2 on p. 46 for a sample reappointment policy) is very similar to the process for initial appointment.

Note: A sample initial appointment policy can be found in Appendix A. In both processes

- the practitioner completes a reapplication request form (see Figure 3. 3 on p. 50 for a sample notification letter and Figure 3.4 for a sample request form)
- the medical staff office gathers and verifies information on the application and collects additional information to determine qualifications and clinical competence
- the appropriate groups and individuals evaluate the collected information and formulate a recommendation
- the governing body, or its appropriate agent, makes a final decision regarding membership reappointment and clinical privileges based on all the results of those reviews

Information collection

When a practitioner reaches his or her reappointment time, collect information about him or her via a reapplication form to assist the appropriate committees in reappraisal.

Information from the practitioner

Reapplications should ask for updated information on a practitioner's

- demographics (e.g., practice location, mailing address, telephone number, etc.)
- external professional activities (i.e., medical association/society memberships)
- affiliations (e.g., medical staff memberships at other hospitals, provider panel memberships with managed care organizations, etc.)
- continuing medical education

Also collect information regarding any current or pending challenges to the practitioner's

- licensure and registration
- membership and clinical privileges at other hospitals, if applicable
- involvement in professional liability actions
- professional society memberships

Hospitals may also choose to evaluate a practitioner's staff category and citizenship, clinical privileges, and health status at reappraisal. See Figure 3.5 on p. 54 for a sample clinical activity summary that reapplicants should review before filling out their reappointment forms.

Information from external sources

Verify a practitioner's claims history (since his or her last appointment) and current coverage directly from the professional liability insurance carrier. Also query the National Practitioner Data Bank (NPDB).

Contact other hospitals about a practitioner's clinical performance only when

- his or her activity level and your internal information is inadequate, as defined by the hospital, to determine current competence
- there is knowledge or suspicion of current, pending, or successful sanctions

Information from internal sources

You can consult your continuously updated credentials filing system or electronic database to gather information about a practitioner's

- licensure
- controlled substance registration (federal and state)
- professional liability insurance coverage
- any other required certifications (e.g., Basic cardiac life support, Advanced cardiac life support

In order for the appropriate committees to evaluate a practitioner's level of compliance with medical staff policies, collect and present for their review internal hospital documents regarding

- meeting attendance
- sanctions imposed/pending
- continuing medical education
- number of admissions/patient care contacts

In addition, pull the practitioner's quality management/reappraisal profile. Collect any peer recommendations (i.e., evaluations from a practitioner within the same medical discipline/specialty).

Review and approval process

When you have collected, verified, and reviewed all of the reappointment data according to the hospital's reappointment policy, compile a summary to use for reappointment decisions. (See Figure 3.36 for a sample summary, on p. 92.) You should then forward the summary and the complete credentials file—including all documentation mentioned above—to the department chair.

Note: The credentials file should be complete before transmitting it to any further party or entity for review.

The department chair makes recommendations to the credentials committee and medical executive committee (MEC) based on the practitioner's staff status, clinical privileges, and clinical performance. From there, the credentials committee and MEC review the department chair's recommendations and forward their recommendations to the hospital governing board for approval or denial.

Record the board's final decision in the credentials file and credentialing database and notify all applicable administrative departments, as well as the practitioner.

Time frames

The elements included in the reappointment process require a significant amount of time and coordination. Depending on the size and complexity of a hospital's medical staff, experience has demonstrated that performing this process for all medical staff members at one time of year does not produce the best results.

To allow focused attention on the production of comparable data, the process should be carried out in a staggered cycle (e.g., quarterly or monthly). Similarly, the reviewing bodies should be given adequate time to focus their attention on comparable inter- and intradepartmental data. For example, hospitals could designate a medical staff year, or appointment period, as the traditional calendar year: January 1–December 31.

Note: This time frame is only a suggestion. Each hospital must decide for itself what makes the most sense.

Establishing a reappointment cycle

Note: Each medical staff member's reappointment cycle is solely determined by the expiration date of his or her current appointment.

When a hospital decides to switch from an annual reappointment cycle to a biennial cycle (i.e., once every two years), it must determine a method for dividing the staff so one half would undergo the reappointment process each year. Most hospitals split the staff in half based on the first initial of the practitioners' last names (i.e., those with last names beginning with A–L or M–Z).

This method of dividing the staff in half should be used only as a means of initiating a two-year reappointment process, not as the method for determining who is reappointed each year thereafter. After all, new members may join the medical staff during various months of the year.

Each new medical staff member must undergo a provisional period for a specified time frame. This time frame must be consistent for all new members. And as stated earlier, the appointment period cannot exceed two years, per JCAHO standard **MS.5.11** (**MS.4.20** in 2004 version).

If a new applicant were reappointed near the end of the cycle based on the first initial of his or her last name, that time period would not be consistent with those of the other medical staff members, and it could exceed the two-year limit.

When membership/clinical privileges are granted, it should be for a specified period of time that includes the "date from" and "date of expiration." Note the definitions below:

- Date from: the date on which the hospital governing board takes final action
- Date of expiration: the date on which the provisional period concludes, *or* the date on which the reappointment cycle concludes (i.e., less than two years from the date on which the governing board took final action)

Defining the time frame

When defining the time frame for reappointment, be sure to allow

- adequate time to prepare reapplication packets (e.g., five months in advance)
- 30 days for receipt of the packet from an individual practitioner
- 60 days for required verification of the practitioner's credentials
- completion of the following reviews based on meeting schedules:
  - Section chief
  - Department chair
  - Any special procedure reviews
  - Credentials committee
  - Executive committee
  - Board of directors

Assembling the reapplication packet

Each practitioner's reapplication packet should include the following items:

- Instruction sheet (see Figure 3.7 on p. 56 for a sample sheet) that
  - explains the reason why the hospital is sending the reapplication
  - lists the items included and instructions for the completion of each
  - gives the time frames for completion and return
  - says whom to call with questions
  - explains the consequences of no response or incomplete response

- Reapplication form (or in lieu of the application form, a reappointment activity profile generated from the credentialing database)
- Questions related to the practitioner's activities outside the hospital, if applicable
- A release statement to provide current consent required for external verification
- Applicable delineation of privilege form from practitioner's previous appointment/reappointment period and a blank privilege request form relevant to his or her clinical area of practice (i.e., general surgery)

Send notification to the following applicable hospital departments from which you need practitioner-specific information for reappraisal:
- Quality management
- Medical records or information services
- Risk management

Provide these departments with a list of individuals in the reappointment cycle and identify what specific information you need. Indicate the time frame for responding with the requested information.

When a practitioner doesn't respond

If the medical staff office does not receive a practitioner's reappointment packet within seven to 14 days following the deadline, send him or her a certified letter (return receipt requested) explaining that failure to fulfill this responsibility results in voluntary termination of membership and clinical privileges when the appointment period expires.

See Figures 3.11 and 3.12 on pp. 66–67 for sample no-response letters.

When a practitioner responds

Upon receipt of a practitioner's reapplication, do the following:

- Date-stamp the information submitted
- Log in the credentials database or on a tracking form the date on which it was received
- Evaluate the information received for completeness
- Send a letter to the practitioner notifying him/her of receipt

For a sample notification letters, see Figures 3.10–3.13 on pp. 65–68.

If any items requested are not received or additional information is required, do either of the following:

- Send a letter to the practitioner requesting missing/additional information
- Notify verbally or via e-mail (be sure to document the notification)

Information to reverify

The following is a rundown of physician information you must reverify upon reappointment.

National Practitioner Data Bank

The Health Care Quality Improvement Act of 1986 requires hospitals to query the NPDB at the time of a practitioner's reappointment.

To query, follow the instructions for using the Integrated Querying and Reporting Service at *www.npdb-hipdb.com*. See also the NPDB *Guidebook* for instructions, which is available for free at the Web site referenced above. The NPDB *Guidebook* reflects the entire range of NPDB policies and operation, including those that have changed or expanded since the NPDB became operational in September 1990. This guidebook is for both new and experienced entities eligible to participate in the NPDB.

State and federal agencies

If a disciplinary or "adverse action" has been taken against a practitioner by a state or federal agency, do the following to obtain information about that action:

- Sending a letter to the applicable agency or log on to the relevant Web sites for information, if applicable
- Obtain the details regarding the action taken and document the source in the practitioner's credentials file
- Check the Department of Health and Human Services' Office of Inspector General Web site for its List of Excluded Individuals and Entities, which documents Medicare and Medicaid sanctions (*http://exclusions.oig.hhs.gov/home.html*)

Malpractice coverage and claims history

Remember to obtain written verification of coverage and claims history from all insurance carriers since the practitioner's last appointment. To all current carriers, send a letter with a release statement, along with a claims history request. Ask the carrier to verify that the practitioner's coverage is applicable to all clinical privileges requested.

To other carriers added since the practitioner's last appointment period, send a letter with a release statements, as well as a request for claims history. (See Figures 3.22–3.23 on pp. 77–78.)

Specialty board certification

If a reapplicant is an MD or DO certified by an American Board of Medical Specialties (ABMS) member board, do the following to verify his or her certification:

- Check in the most recent edition of The Official ABMS Directory of Board Certified Medical Specialists (an annual compendium of all ABMS board-certified practitioners available in book, CD/ROM, or online format)
- Call the ABMS directly at 866/ASK-ABMS
- Document findings on the "Verification of specialty board certification status" form (see Figure 3.25 on p. 80) and file it in the reapplicant's credentials file
- Obtain original certification documentation from the respective member board
- Obtain updated verification directly from the respective member board

If a practitioner is an osteopath, dentist, podiatrist, or MD certified by a non-ABMS board, verify the board's recognition with the applicable national society send a letter to the applicable board requesting verification of specialty board status

Note: The certification requirements of non-ABMS boards should be evaluated.

Additional training

To verify additional formal professional training since the last appointment, send a letter to the program director and/or the individual who provided direct supervision. In the letter, request verification of the training and a performance evaluation. (See Figures 3.26–3.39 on pp. 81–98.)

Other primary hospital affiliations

If a practitioner's activity level is below the level your hospital has deemed necessary for evaluating current competence, contact the clinical department chair at the hospital(s) where he or she is active and obtain a performance/clinical competence evaluation.

Send a letter to this/these hospital(s) requesting this information, and include verification form. (See Figures 3.31–3.34 on pp. 87–90.)

Preparing information for review

Compile the information they collect from the reapplicant and from internal and external sources for the review process (see Figure 3.36 on p. 92). From it, an evaluation can be conducted and a judgment can be made.

The following are the basic elements required that you should compile for each reapplicant:

- An administrative profile that includes the
  - name and professional title
  - date of initial appointment
  - date of last appointment and appointment expiration
  - date current reappointment period (make sure to state to and from dates)
  - current and requested staff status
  - current department/division affiliation
  - current certification status
- Information from practitioner, including
  - current office address(s)
  - self-declared specialty/specialties
  - practice affiliation(s)
  - additional formal professional training
  - current faculty appointments
  - current hospital affiliations
  - changes in certification status
  - evaluation of health status
  - any additional data needed for clarification purposes
- Relative information and verification from external sources
- Administrative data related to this reappointment period, including
  - medico-administrative positions held
  - attendance
  - committee meetings
  - clinical department/section meetings
  - continuing medical education conferences (if required)

Committee review process

Once all of the pertinent information is compiled, the reapplication is brought before the appropriate department chair, credentials committee, MEC, and finally, the governing board for their review and approval.

Peer recommendations

Peer recommendations are part of the basis for developing recommendations for continued medical staff membership and/or the delineation of clinical privileges. Peers are defined as those with the same professional education and background as the applicant. For example, a physician evaluates a physician; a dentist evaluates a dentist; a podiatrist evaluates a podiatrist.

If the department chair is not in the applicant's peer group, a written recommendation must be obtained from one of the applicant's peers. This peer should be a medical staff member who is capable of evaluating the information obtained from the hospital's quality monitoring. Or it can be an individual who is a peer, but not a member of the staff, who has direct information regarding the practitioner's current clinical competence.

Department chair

The department chair must perform an evaluation of the practitioner's performance and make recommendations for reappointment and clinical privileges based on that evaluation. (See Figure 3.35 for a sample department chair report and recommendations on p. 91.) This evaluation must include confirmation of the applicant's declaration of health status. Provide the department chair with a complete practitioner profile that meets the essential elements (as previously outlined), including applicable peer recommendations.

Credentials committee

The credentials committee reviews the credentials file and reapplication to ensure that the administrative and departmental review processes are in step with outlined procedures. This committee also evaluates the reapplicant's privilege(s) request and makes recommendations to the MEC for reappointment and clinical privileges. The credentials committee receives an agenda listing the candidates for reappointment categorized as follows (under each category, the candidates should be listed by department and alphabetized by last name):

1. Same status and same privileges
2. Status/privileges increased
3. Status/privileges decreased

For categories 2 and 3, practitioners' profiles should be available for the committee and used as appropriate.

Medical executive committee

Once a reapplication has moved through the credentials committee, it goes to the MEC for its review and recommendation. As in the initial appointment process, the MEC may choose to forward the credentials committee's recommendation as its own. If the credentials committee's recommendation is deemed adverse, the applicant has the right to request a fair hearing.

Governing body

After the MEC, the reapplication goes before the governing body for a final review and action. The medical staff office should inform the practitioner and applicable individuals about the final action. See Figures 3.42–3.44 on pp. 105–107 for sample notification letters. The board's activities in the reappointment stage follow the final steps as outlined in the medical staff bylaws and the initial appointment policy. See the Appendix A, p. 237, for a sample initial appointment policy.

Do's and don'ts for the department chair, credentials committee, and MEC

Don't

✗ review the reapplication file until all necessary information has been collected and verified. In other words, don't try to guess or assume anything—insist on accurate and verified information confirming both qualifications and current clinical competence.

✗ give in to peer or administrative pressure to review a reapplication prematurely or hastily.

✗ assume all physicians are entitled to reappointment unless proven incompetent.

✗ worry unduly about legal action. Remember, the board makes the final decision; the department chair, credentials committee, and MEC roles are advisory.

✗ hesitate to table a reapplication that warrants further investigation.

Do

✓ review reapplications with a medical staff services professional, as he or she knows the files well.

✓ ask yourself, "If this practitioner is reappointed by the board, would I be comfortable referring a neighbor to him or her?"

✓ recognize that ongoing performance monitoring is the very best way to avoid any surprises at reappointment

✓ make sure the institution has agreed, through insurance or indemnification, to protect the committees in case a physician should file a lawsuit.

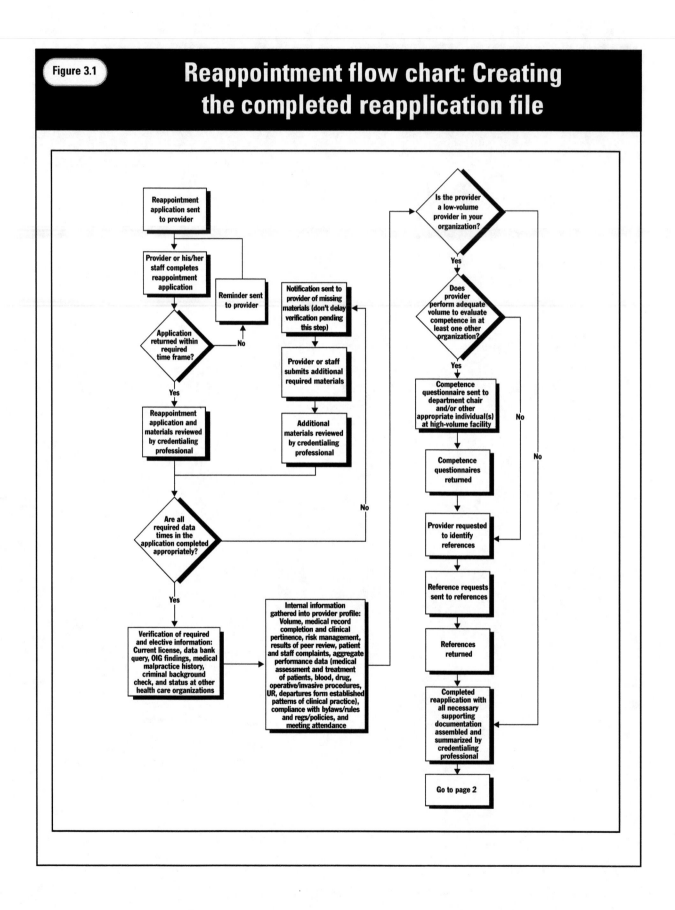

Figure 3.1

Reappointment flow chart: Creating the completed reapplication file

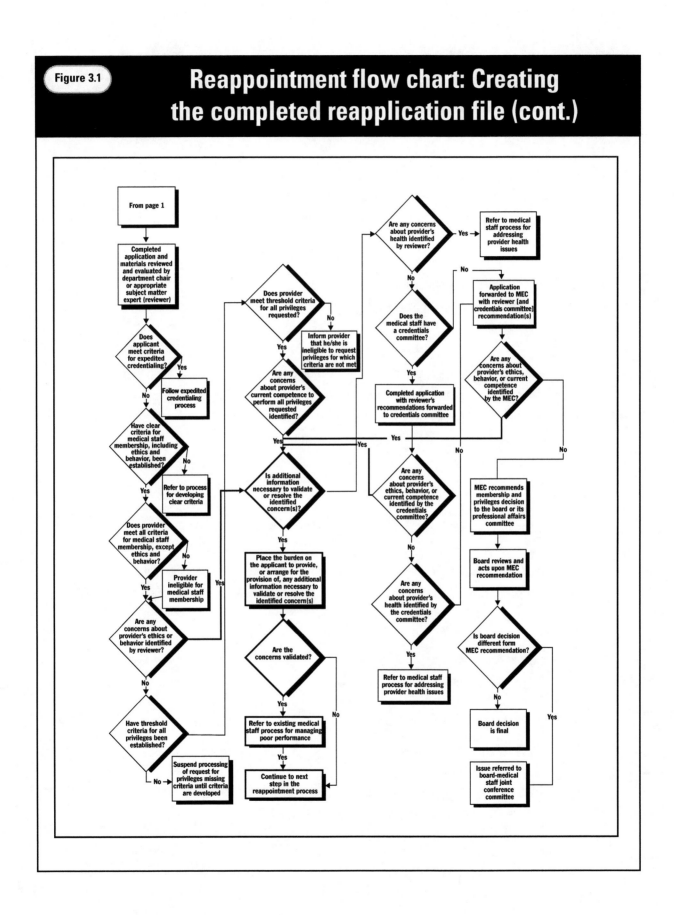

Figure 3.1

Reappointment flow chart: Creating the completed reapplication file (cont.)

| Figure 3.2 | **Reappointment policy** |

Policy

All appointments (except provisional) are for a period not to exceed two years. At least three months before the expiration date of a medical staff appointment, the chief executive officer or his designee will notify the appointee of the date of expiration and supply him or her with an application for reappointment packet.

Information collection and verification

From appointees: At least 60 days before the expiration date of his or her appointment, the appointee shall provide the hospital with the following information:

- Complete information to update his or her file on items listed in his or her original application
- Continuing training and education external to the hospital during the preceding period
- Specific request for the clinical privileges sought on reappointment, with any basis for changes
- Requests for changes in staff category or department assignments

If the appointee fails, without good cause, to provide this information, the hospital will deem the failure a voluntary resignation from the medical staff, and the appointment will automatically expire unless the credentials committee explicitly extends the appointment for not more than two 30-day periods.

The medical staff office will verify this additional information and notify the appointee of any inadequacies in the information or verification problems. The appointee will have the burden of producing adequate information and resolving any doubts about the data.

From internal/external sources: The medical staff office will collect the following information regarding the appointee's professional and collegial activities:

- Currency of licensure and registrations
- Professional board certification status
- Any pending or completed disciplinary actions or sanctions
- Performance and conduct in this hospital/other health care organizations, including his or her
    - patterns of care as demonstrated in findings of quality
    - assessment/performance improvement activities

| Figure 3.2 | **Reappointment policy (cont.)** |

- clinical judgment and skills in the treatment of patients
- behavior and cooperation with hospital personnel, patients, and visitors
- medical records/hospital reports completion
- satisfactory completion of 40 hours of continuing medical education activities
- attendance at required medical staff and department meetings
- service on medical staff, department, and hospital committees
- timely and accurate completion of medical records
- compliance with all applicable bylaws, policies, rules, regulations, and procedures of the hospital and staff

The hospital shall review and verify the above information according to the initial appointment policy.

The medical staff coordinator will compile a summary of clinical activity at this hospital for each appointee due for reappointment.

Procedure for processing applications for reappointment

The medical staff office shall notify the quality improvement department of the need to collect all pertinent medical staff committee minutes and studies and to prepare a summary of findings for the appointee.

The medical staff office shall send the complete file, including all documentation mentioned above, to the chair of each department in which the staff appointee requests or has exercised privileges.

Department action: Each appropriate department chair will review the appointee's file as described above and forward to the credentials committee a written report of the appointee's performance, including the following:

- A statement as to whether he or she knows of, has observed, or has been informed of any conduct that indicates significant present or potential physical or behavioral problems that affect the practitioner's ability to perform professional and medical staff duties appropriately[1]
- Recommendations regarding

---

[1] *Health care organizations must comply with the Americans with Disabilities Act.*

Figure 3.2 — Reappointment policy (cont.)

- Reappointment
- Staff category
- Department assignment
- Clinical privileges

Credentials committee action: The credentials committee will review the appointee's file, department reports, and all other relevant information and forward to the MEC a written report with recommendations regarding the following:

- Reappointment,
- Staff category
- Department assignment
- Clinical privileges

The credentials committee will follow the decision process outlined in the Initial Appointment Policy.

MEC action: The MEC will review the appointee's file, the department report(s), credentials committee report(s), and all relevant information available to it and forward to the board a written report with recommendations for the following:

- Reappointment
- Staff category
- Department assignment
- Clinical privileges

The MEC shall follow the decision process outlined in the Initial Appointment Policy. If the MEC's recommendation is deemed adverse, no such adverse recommendation will be forwarded to the board until after the practitioner has exercised or has waived his or her right to a hearing as provided in the medical staff bylaws.

Figure 3.2 — Reappointment policy (cont.)

Final processing and governing board action: To complete processing of the application, the hospital shall follow the procedures in the Initial Appointment Policy with the following changes:

- An "adverse recommendation" by the board will mean a recommendation or action to
  - deny reappointment
  - deny a requested change in the appointee's staff category or department assignment
  - change, without the staff appointee's consent, his or her staff category or department assignment
  - deny or restrict requested clinical privileges

- The terms "applicant" and "appointment," as used in these sections, shall be read respectively, as "appointee" and "reappointment"

Figure 3.3 — Notification letter to practitioner regarding reappointment

Dear Dr. _____:

  Appointee

As you know, medical staff appointments are for a two-year period. Your current appointment and clinical privileges are about to expire. The reappointment process is outlined in the hospital's credentialing policy and procedure manual.

Enclosed with this packet of materials is a brief medical staff reappointment request and information form for you to complete if you wish to be reappointed to the medical staff of this hospital. Also included are a new request for clinical privileges form and a list of your current clinical privileges, including the number of times you have exercised each privilege within this reappointment period. When reviewing your current privileges list, and completing the new privilege request forms, please keep in mind your current clinical practice pattern.

If you have not used a privilege in several years, you might wish to voluntarily relinquish the privilege. Otherwise, you might be asked to supply your department chair with evidence of training, continuing education or proficiency. Any requests for new or increased privileges must be accompanied by information demonstrating current clinical competence in the privileges requested. Information should be supplied in original form, (e.g., certificates, continuing medical education credits) demonstrating education, training, and experience you believe qualifies you for the privilege(s). In addition, one letter from a recognized expert in the clinical discipline involved should be submitted.

Please review and update the information on the attached form (or profile) and answer all questions, complete the applicable forms and return them to the medical staff office as soon as possible, but no later than 30 days from this date. If you have any questions or need any assistance, please do not hesitate to contact the medical staff office or me.

Thank you for your cooperation. We look forward to your continued participation in the hospital's mission.

Sincerely,

Chief executive officer
Enclosures

Figure 3.4

Reappointment request and information form

For medical staff office use:

Date form sent: _____ Date form received: _____

Name: _____

Expiration date of current appointment: _____

Department/section assignment: _____
❏ Active   ❏ Associate   ❏ Courtesy

1. Do you wish to be reappointed to the medical staff of this hospital?   ❏ Yes   ❏ No

2. Please complete a new privilege request form for the desired privileges (see attached copy of your
   current privileges) and add or delete according to your current clinical practice patterns. Please note:
   All requests for additional or modification of clinical privileges must be accompanied by information
   documenting training, experience and current clinical competence.

3. Please submit a copy of your current state license, Drug Enforcement Administration (DEA) permit
   and professional liability insurance face sheet or other evidence of current coverage for the privileges
   you are requesting.

   If you answer yes to any of the following questions, please provide an explanation on the reverse
   side of this form or on a separate sheet of paper and attach.

4. Since your last reappointment:

   Has your license (MD, DO, DDS, DMD, DPM, PhD) in any jurisdiction ever been
   challenged, limited, suspended, or revoked, or is your license currently subject
   to any successful or pending challenge?   ❏ Yes   ❏ No

   Has your DEA number ever been limited, suspended, or revoked, or is it currently subject to any successfully or pending challenge?   ❏ Yes   ❏ No

Figure 3.4

Reappointment request and information form (cont.)

Have your privileges at any hospital ever been suspended, diminished, revoked, or not renewed? ❏ Yes ❏ No

Has your specialty board status ever been suspended or revoked? ❏ Yes ❏ No

Have you taken an examination for board certification and failed since your last appointment/reappointment? ❏ Yes ❏ No

Have you ever been denied appointment, or clinical privileges, or renewal thereof, or been subject to disciplinary action by any medical staff/hospital, or resigned from a medical staff? ❏ Yes ❏ No

Have you been named in a malpractice action within the past five years? ❏ Yes ❏ No

Has your faculty appointment or membership in any medical or other professional school ever not been renewed or subject to disciplinary action? ❏ Yes ❏ No

Have you ever requested a fair hearing or board appeal? ❏ Yes ❏ No

Have you ever brought litigation against a hospital or medical staff? ❏ Yes ❏ No

Have you received any type of sanction from a professional review organization (PRO), or third-party payer including a state/federal or regulatory agency? ❏ Yes ❏ No

Have you ever been denied appointment or clinical privileges, or renewal thereof, or have you ever voluntarily relinquished clinical privileges or resigned from a medical staff? ❏ Yes ❏ No

Is any such action or investigation pending? ❏ Yes ❏ No

Figure 3.4

Reappointment request and information form (cont).

5. Have you had any recent physical, mental, or behavioral problems that might affect your ability to safely treat patients at this hospital?[1] ❑ Yes ❑ No

If yes, please explain below or on the reverse side of this form or on a separate sheet of paper and attach:

_____

_____

_____

_____

Regardless of how this question is answered, the application will be processed in the usual manner. If you have answered this question affirmatively and are found to be professionally qualified for medical staff appointment and the clinical privileges requested, you will be given an opportunity to meet with the physician's health task force to determine what accommodations are necessary or feasible to allow you to continue to practice safely.

6. Since your last appointment, have you joined any other hospital staff or health care organization? ❑ Yes ❑ No

If yes, please list below:

_____

_____

_____

_____

I hereby request reappointment to the medical staff of this hospital with requested clinical privileges as shown on the attached. I acknowledge that I have been given access to the medical staff's current bylaws, rules and regulations and hospital policies, and hereby agree to abide by them.

_____   _____

Applicant's signature   Date

---

[1] All health care organizations must follow the Americans with Disabilities Act.

Figure 3.5 | **Current clinical activity**

Name _____ Period of Review: From __/__/__/ to __/__/__/___

Department _____ Clinical specialty _____

Dear Dr. _____:
            [insert practitioner name]

Below is a list of your current clinical privileges taken from your credentials file and the volume of activity information related to those privileges.

Privilege   **Number of times treated/performed**

_____   _____

_____   _____

_____   _____

_____   _____

_____   _____

_____   _____

_____   _____

_____   _____

_____   _____

_____   _____

_____   _____

_____   _____

_____   _____

_____   _____

_____   _____

Please review this list in preparation for completing the attached new request for clinical privileges and indicate any corrections, deletions, and additions, relevant to your current clinical practice patterns.

Please note: All requests for increased or new clinical privileges must be accompanied by information demonstrating current clinical competence in the privileges requested. Information should be supplied (original form) demonstrating the education, training, and experience you believe qualifies you for the privileges requested. In addition, one letter from a recognized expert in the clinical discipline involved should be submitted.

Figure 3.6

Request for modification of clinical privileges

Note: All requests for increased privileges must be accompanied by information demonstrating current clinical competence in the privileges requested. Information should be supplied (original form) demonstrating the education, training, and experience you believe qualifies you for the privileges. You should submit at least one letter from a recognized expert in the clinical discipline involved as well.

I hereby request additional clinical privileges as follows (or see attached).

A. _____

B. _____

C. _____

D. _____

E. _____

I have attached full details demonstrating my competence in these areas.

_____

_____

Print name _____

Signature _____

Date _____

| Figure 3.7 | Instructions for completion of application for reappointment |

You must complete and return the following by: *[date]*

Reappointment profile:
The enclosed profile shows current information on file. *(See attached.)*

- Update and/or correct the information directly on profile.
- If there is not sufficient space on the profile, include attachments.
- If you are requesting a change in staff status, indicate the requested change directly on the form.
- Complete the listing of all continuing medical education (CME) programs that you attended since your last reappointment with the credits earned, or attach copies.
- Answer questions about disciplinary action and clinical performance, and complete the section on professional liability insurance, as applicable.
- Sign and date the terms and conditions of reappointment; return the form together with the privilege request form and your reapplication fee of *[dollar amount]*.

Clinical privileges request:
You must submit a new clinical privileges request form. Enclosed is a new listing of all privileges in your specialty. Below each specific privilege, your current status is indicated (i.e., granted, not requested, denied).

- Complete the clinical privileges request form for your specific specialty.
- Sign, date, and return the privileges request form.
- If you are requesting new privilege(s) for procedure(s) never requested or granted at *[insert hospital name]*, you must attach documentation of training and/or experience with the requests.
- If you are deleting or not requesting a privilege you held during the past reappointment cycle, please indicate the reason for it.

Release forms:
- Sign, date, and return the terms and conditions of reappointment form and the professional liability insurance release form.

Return the complete packet to:
[Contact name]
[Hospital name]
[Hospital address]

If you have any questions, please call:
Medical staff office
[Phone number]

Figure 3.8 — Reappointment profile for individual practitioners

01/26/03
[Hospital name]
P. 1
Date: 6/01/01 **thru:** 1/26/03

Name: Doe, John Q.
Date of birth: 7/04/50
Home address: 123 Any Street
Anytown, NY 01234

Practitioner category: MD
Citizenship: USA
Phone: 123-456-7890

Office name: General Surgery, Inc.
123 Main Street
Anytown, NY 01234

Phone: 111-222-3333
Answering service: 222-333-444

Mailing address: General Surgery, Inc.
123 Main Street
Anytown, NY 01234

Practice type: Solo
Requested staff category: Active
Current staff category: Active
Initial appointment: 7/01/91
Appointment expires: 6/30/01

Leaves: Provisional periods for status privileges changes

Specialty: General surgery
(GS)
Vascular surgery
(VS)

Current:	Department(s)	Section(s)	Member
	Surgery	GS	Y
	Surgery	VS	Y

Requested:	Department(s)	Section(s)	Member
	Surg	GS	Y

License(s):	MD	MA	#765897	Exp: 6/30/04
Restrictions:		None		

Figure 3.8 — Reappointment profile for individual practitioners (cont.)

01/26/03
[Hospital name]
P. 2
Date: 6/01/01 **thru:** 1/26/03

Name: Doe, John Q.   **Practitioner category:** MD

Controlled substance permit(s):

    NY   #ADA-00-123456   Exp: 6/30/04

Inc. category: II III IV V-A V-B
    US   #JOH-01-123456   Exp: 6/30/04

Other graduate education:

    Harvard School of Public Health   6/86   Boston, MA

Other postgraduate training: VASC SURG
11/87-01/88   Massachusetts General Hospital

Board certification in: GS
By: American Board of Surgery   Exp: *[insert date]*

Other certification: Nd/YAG laser for general surgery
By: Bremer   Exp: *[insert date]*

Hospital affiliations:

    09/90-   Central Medical Center   Consulting
    04/91-   St. Mary's Hospital   Consulting
    09/90-   Emmaus House   Board member

Other institutional affiliations:

    08/91   Primary Care Physician, Inc. Consultant
    05/89-   United Physicians PHO   Medical director

Academic appointments:

    07/89-12/90   Syracuse University
                  Surgery   Clinical associate

Figure 3.8 — Reappointment profile for individual practitioners (cont.)

01/26/03
[Hospital name]
P. 3
Date: 6/01/01 **thru:** 1/26/03

Name: Doe, John Q.

Practitioner category: MD

Professional and community memberships:

American College of Surgeons
American Heart Association
American Cancer Society
New York Surgical Society

Med Group Mgmt Assn
New York Medical Society
Society of Critical Care Medicine

Insurance carrier:
Limits:
Exclusions:

Metro Insurance Company
$1,000,000/$3,000,000 From: 6/01/90 Exp: 5/31/03
None

Claims/suits activity:

	Current period	Prior 3 years	Next prior 5 years
	0	0	1
	1	0	0
	1	0	1

Sanctions/problems:

In current period: 1
In prior years: 0
In next prior 5 years: 0

Continuing education:

	Hours
12/03/01-12/05/01	12 Nd-YAG laser in surgery Chicago, IL
10/31/02-11/02/02	12 Hyperalimentation in SICU patients San Francisco, CA

In-house continuing education:

	Hours	
5/12/02-5/13/02	10	Basic life support
12/12/02-12/12/02	3	The Health Care Quality Improvement Act
2/03/95-2/03/95	3	Developments in hyperalimentation
8/02/02-8/02/02	4	New drugs for basic medical problems
2/01/02-2/01/03	4	Advances in respiratory care

Meeting attendance:

	Held	Attended	Excused	%
General staff	8	4	2	75
SURG	5	5	0	100
Credentials	2	1	1	100
Pharmacy and therapeutics	2	1	0	50

Figure 3.8

Reappointment profile for individual practitioners (cont.)

01/26/03
[Hospital name]
P. 4
Date: 6/01/01 **thru:** 1/26/03

Name: Doe, John Q.   **Practitioner category:** M.D.

Other events:	Total		Yes		%
Dues	1		1		100
Medacknowl	1		1		100
On-call	1		1		100
Reapplica	1		1		100
Teach	2		2		100

Medical record suspension: #:1   **Total days:** 2

Administrative positions:

01/95-12/96	President elect of general medical staff
01/96-12/97	Committee chair of medical quality review committee
12/96-	Committee chair of surgical quality review committee
01/97-12/99	Section head of general surgery
01/99-12/01	Department chair of surgery

Figure 3.9

General surgery clinical privileges

Name: _____

☐ Initial appointment   ☐ Reappointment
☐ Effective from __/__/__ to __/__/__

All new applicants must meet the following requirements as approved by the Board of Trustees effective: __/__/__

Qualifications

Current certification or active participation in the examination process leading to certification in general surgery by the American Board of Surgery, or the American Osteopathic Board of Surgery.

Or

Successful completion of an ACGME- or AOA-accredited post-graduate training program in general surgery.

Required previous experience

Applicant must be able to demonstrate performance of at least 100 general surgical procedures during the past 12 months or demonstrate successful participation in a hospital-affiliated formalized residency or special clinical fellowship.

Special procedures

Successful completion of an approved, recognized course when such exists, or acceptable supervised training in residency, fellowship or other acceptable experience, and documentation of competence to obtain and retain clinical privileges as set forth in medical staff policies governing the exercise of specific privileges.

Reappointment requirements

Current demonstrated competence and an adequate volume of current experience with acceptable results in the privileges requested for the past 24 months based on results of quality assessment/improvement activities and outcomes.

Note: If any privileges are covered by an exclusive contractual agreement, physicians who are not a party to the contract are not eligible to request the privilege(s), regardless of education, training and experience.

Figure 3.9

General surgery clinical privileges (cont.)

Name: _____

❑ Initial appointment   ❑ Reappointment
❑ Effective from __/__/__ to __/__/__

Applicant: Check off the "Requested" box for each privilege requested. New applicants may be requested to provide documentation of the number and types of hospital cases during the past 24 months. Applicants have the burden of producing information deemed adequate by the Hospital for a proper evaluation of current competence, and other qualifications and for resolving any doubts.

Department chair/chief: Check the appropriate box for recommendation on the last page of this form. If recommended with conditions or not recommended, provide condition or explanation on the last page of this form.

GENERAL SURGERY CORE PRIVILEGES
❑ **Requested**

> Admit, evaluate, diagnose, consult, and provide pre-, intra-, and post-operative care, and perform surgical procedures to patients of all ages, except where specifically excluded from practice; correct or treat various conditions, diseases, disorders, and injuries of the alimentary tract, abdomen, and its contents, extremities, breast, skin and soft tissue, head and neck, vascular, and endocrine systems. Management of trauma and complete care of critically ill patients with underlying surgical conditions in the emergency department, intensive care unit, and trauma/burn units. The attached procedure list reflects the scope of practice included in this core.

Special procedures or techniques
(See qualifications and/or specific criteria)

USE OF LASER
❑ **Requested**

> Requires: Completion of an approved eight-hour minimum continuing medical education (CME) course that includes training in laser principles and safety, basic laser physics, laser tissue interaction, discussions of the clinical specialty field, and hands-on experience with lasers. A letter outlining the content and successful completion of course must be submitted, or documentation of successful completion of an approved residency in a specialty or subspecialty that included training in laser principles and safety, basic laser physics, laser tissue interaction, discussions of the clinical specialty field, and a minimum of six hours of observation and hands-on experience with lasers.

LAPAROSCOPIC NISSEN FUNDOPLICATION (ANTIREFLUX SURGERY)
❑ **Requested**

> Requires: Successful completion of an accredited residency in general surgery that included advanced laparoscopic training; a formal course in laparoscopic Nissen fundoplication that included preceptorship by a surgeon experience in the procedure; and performance of at least 25 laparoscopic Nissen fundoplication procedures in the past 12 months. ***Maintenance of privilege:*** Requires performance of at least 10 laparoscopic Nissen fundoplication procedures in the past 12 months.

Figure 3.9 **General surgery clinical privileges (cont.)**

Name: _____

❑ Effective from __/__/__ to __/__/__

STEREOTACTIC BREAST BIOPSY
❑ **Requested**

Requires: Successful completion of training in the stereotactic and ultrasound-guided technique of breast biopsy during residency or in an accredited course or institution; and possession of privileges for breast imaging interpretation. Required previous experience: Successful completion of at least 15 hours of Category 1 CME in stereotactic breast biopsy or performance of at least 36 stereotactic breast biopsies in the past three years; successful evaluation of at least 480 mammograms per year in the last two years in consultation with a physician who is qualified to interpret mammography under the Mammography Quality Standards Act of 1992 (MQSA); successful completion of at least four hours of Category 1 continuing medical education in medical radiation physics; and performance of either of the following: At least 12 stereotactic breast biopsies; or at least three hands-on procedures with a physician who is qualified to interpret mammography under the MQSA and has performed at least 24 procedures. Maintenance of privilege: Performance of at least 12 stereotactic breast biopsies in the past 12 months.

BARIATRIC SURGERY (STOMACH STAPLING) FOR MORBID OBESITY
❑ **Requested**

Requires: Successful completion of an accredited residency in general surgery and a preceptorship in open an/or laparoscopic bariatric surgery. Required previous experience: Performance of at least 20 procedures in the past 12 months. Maintenance of privilege: Performance of at least 20 surgical open or laparoscopic bariatric procedures annually.

SENTINEL LYMPH NODE BIOPSY FOR BREAST CANCER
❑ **Requested**

Requires: Successful completion of an accredited residency in general surgery and proficiency in the standard diagnosis and surgical management of breast cancer. Required previous experience: Successful completion of an approved course leading to the ability to evaluate the patient for the sentinel node mapping procedure, understand the clinical implications of the findings, and become familiar with the technique and equipment used. Note: It is recommended that if the physician performing sentinel lymph node biopsy for breast cancer does not have direct training or experience in both nuclear medicine and pathology, then the physician must have access to individuals who have expertise in those areas.

ADMINISTRATION OF MODERATE CONSCIOUS SEDATION IN ACCORDANCE WITH HOSPITAL POLICY
❑ **Requested**

Figure 3.9 — General surgery clinical privileges (cont.)

Name: _____

❏ Initial appointment
❏ Reappointment
❏ Effective from __/__/__ to __/__/__

Acknowledgement of practitioner

I have requested only those privileges for which by education, training, current experience and demonstrated performance I am qualified to perform and for which I wish to exercise at [insert hospital name], and I understand that:

(a) In exercising any clinical privileges granted, I am constrained by hospital and medical staff policies and rules applicable generally and any applicable to the particular situation.

(b) Any restriction on the clinical privileges granted to me is waived in an emergency situation and in such situation my actions are governed by the applicable section of the medical staff bylaws or related documents.

Signed: _____ Date: _____

Department Chair's Recommendation

I have reviewed the requested clinical privileges and supporting documentation for the above-named applicant and make the following recommendation(s):

❏ Recommend all requested privileges
❏ Recommend privileges with the following conditions/modifications:
❏ Do not recommend the following requested privileges:

Privilege	Condition/modification/explanation
1.	
2.	
3.	
Notes:	

Department chair signature: _____ Date: _____

Credentials committee chair signature: _____ Date: _____

MEC action: _____ Date: _____

Board of trustee's action: _____ Date: _____

Figure 3.10 — Notification of receipt of reapplication

[Date]

Dear [Name]:

We received your reappointment application and request for continuation of clinical privileges.

We will do an initial check of the reapplication for completeness and consistency, notify you if necessary about any additional information required, and then begin the process of verifying the information provided on the reapplication.

Thank you for your promptness in returning the reapplication. We look forward to your continued participation in [hospital name]'s medical staff.

Sincerely,

[Vice president of medical affairs]

Figure 3.11 No response to request for additional information

[Date]

Dear [Name]:

The period within which you were supposed to respond to our request for additional information or clarification on your application for reappointment and clinical privileges has now ended. We have not received your reply. We take your non-response as an indication that you wish to voluntarily relinquish your appointment and privileges as of [appointment expiration date].

Accordingly, we have terminated any further review of your reappraisal and consider the file closed. Except as provided in the next paragraph of this letter, the file may be reopened only as provided in the medical staff bylaws.

If unpredictable, extenuating circumstances prevented you from making a timely response to the request and from notifying us prior to the deadline of your inability to do so, please send a full written explanation of those facts to my attention in the medical staff office within 10 days of the date of this letter, along with the additional information or clarification originally requested. If this explanation is satisfactory to the applicable hospital representatives, processing of your reappointment will resume at the point at which it was suspended.

Any failure to respond according to the terms of this paragraph will have the same effect as the failure to respond to the original request, except without any opportunity to reopen the matter as provided in this paragraph.

Sincerely,

[President and chief executive officer]

Enclosures

Figure 3.12

No response resulting in voluntary relinquishment of appointment and privileges

[Date]

Dear *[Name]*:

According to the medical staff bylaws, appointment to the medical staff of *[hospital name]* lasts for a period of no more than two years, per the special conditions of each individual's appointment. The procedures for reappointment require the practitioner whose appointment is expiring to provide certain information to the medical staff office.

Since your current appointment expires on *[expiration date]*, a request letter (dated *[letter date]*) was sent asking you to complete and return the necessary forms. The deadline set forth in that letter for returning the forms has now passed. As specified in the medical staff bylaws, this failure constitutes a voluntary relinquishment of your medical staff appointment and clinical privileges effective on the expiration of your current appointment.

If you have any questions regarding this matter, please contact me at [*phone number*].

Sincerely,

[President and chief executive officer]

Figure 3.13

Notification of receipt of reapplication and required additional information

[Date]

Dear [Name]:

We have received your reappointment application, request for clinical privileges, and related materials. Initial check and review of the materials indicate that additional information or clarification is necessary on particular items.

The specific information or explanation required is detailed in the attachment to this letter.

Within 30 days from the date of this letter, please send a written reply to my attention in the medical staff office, providing accurate and complete information in response to this request. The processing of your reapplication will resume as soon as we receive a satisfactory reply. If we do not receive a reply by the deadline noted, we will consider it an indication that you do not wish to continue your medical staff membership and exercise your clinical privileges when they expire.

Please contact me if you have any questions. Thank you for your cooperation in this matter.

Sincerely,

[Manager, medical staff office]

Enclosure

Figure 3.14 | Notification of receipt of requested information

[Date]

Dear *[Name]*:

We have received your reply to our letter requesting information or clarification regarding your application for reappointment and clinical privileges.

Review of the application through the appropriate channels will now resume.

Thank you for your cooperation.

Sincerely,

[Manager, medical staff office]

Figure 3.15   Request for further clarification or information

[Date]

Dear *[Name]*:

We received your reply to our letter requesting additional information or clarification of your application for reappointment and clinical privileges. Upon reviewing it, we did not find that it fully responded to the request. If you misunderstood or misinterpreted our initial request, let us clarify it.

The reasons for which we deemed your initial reply nonresponsive, and the exact information required to satisfactorily respond to the request, are detailed in the attachment to this letter.

As soon as possible, but no more than 10 days from the date of this letter, please send accurate, complete information, in writing, in response to this inquiry the medical staff office. Processing of your application for reappointment will resume as soon as we receive your reply. If we do not receive a reply by the deadline provided, we will consider it an indication that you do not wish to continue your appointment or exercise your clinical privileges when they expire.

Thank you for your cooperation in this matter.

Sincerely,

[Manager, credentialing services]
Enclosure

Figure 3.16

Verification process
for reappointment/reappraisal

QUERY NATIONAL PRACTITIONER
DATA BANK

STATE LICENSURE AND STATE ——————▶ If individual maintains license/
CONTROLLED SUBSTANCE practice in other state(s)
REGISTRATION • Written with state regarding
current sanctions

▼

Problem/sanction identified
• Written information
• Obtained from state

ADDITIONAL POSTGRADUATE ——————▶ U.S./Canadian only
SINCE LAST REAPPOINTMENT • Written
- Attendance
- Competence
- Problems

CHANGES IN HOSPITAL/INSTITUTIONAL/ ——————▶ U.S./Canadian only
ORGANIZATIONAL AFFILIATIONS • Written
(including academic, managed care, and practice) - Competence
- Problems

IF INACTIVE AT THIS HOSPITAL, ALL ——————▶ U.S./Canadian only
CURRENT ORGANIZATIONAL • Written
AFFILIATIONS (including academic, - Competence
managed care, and practice) - Problems

PROFESSIONAL LIABILITY ——————▶ Current carrier ——————▶ Carriers since reappointment
COVERAGE AND CLAIMS HISTORY • Current coverage • Coverage periods
• Claims history • Claims history
• Lapses/discontinuation

CHANGES IN SPECIALTY ——————▶ If certified ——————▶ Certification/qualification expired
CERTIFICATION • ABMS member board • Written with board
- ABMS annual publication
- ABMS 800#
- AOA member board
- AOA div. cert.
• ADA/APMA-recognized board
- Written with board
• Nonmember/recognized board
- Written with board
- Also obtain board requirements

PEER RECOMMENDATIONS ——————▶ Internal as part of review ——————▶ If no knowledgeable
and recommendation process peers on staff
• Reference required
- Written competence
- Health status

Figure 3.17 — Verification of licensure

[Date]

Re: [Name]
    State:
    Type of license:
    License #:

Dear Sir/Madam:

The above-named practitioner has applied for reappointment to the [hospital name] medical staff and for continuation of clinical privileges.

The application indicates licensure in your jurisdiction as described above. We would appreciate your verifying this license and providing us with other specific information regarding the applicant. To do so, please complete the attached form and return it to us in the enclosed envelope. A prompt and full reply will be appreciated.

Also enclosed is a copy of a signed release and immunity statement. This statement constitutes consent to this inquiry and to your response, and releases from liability any individual who provides the requested information.

Thank you for your cooperation.

Sincerely,

[Manager, credentialing services]
Enclosures

Figure 3.18

Verification of licensure and disciplinary proceedings

Re: *[Practitioner's full name]*
    Time period under review:
    State/type of license:
    License #:

Above license/certificate number correct?   ❑ Yes   ❑ No

If no, correct number is: _____

Date issued: _____ Date expires: _____

If any of the following questions are answered with "Yes," please provide full details on a separate sheet.

1. Has the practitioner voluntarily relinquished or limited his license to practice during the time period under review indicated above?   ❑ Yes   ❑ No

2. Has the board revoked, suspended, reduced, limited, made probationary, or not renewed the practitioner's license certificate during said time period?   ❑ Yes   ❑ No

3. Was any proceeding initiated by the board that could have resulted in any of the actions indicated in #2 above, during said time period, or is any such proceeding pending?   ❑ Yes   ❑ No

4. Did any health care institution, practitioner, or other entity or agency report taking any professional sanctions against the practitioner or other circumstances that may be pertinent to our credentialing process during that period?   ❑ Yes   ❑ No

5. Did any entity report to you that it made a payment for the benefit of the practitioner in settlement (or partial settlement) of or in satisfaction of a judgment in a medical malpractice action or claim during that time period?   ❑ Yes   ❑ No

Verified and completed by: _____

Name (type or print): _____ Title: _____

Signature: _____ Date: _____

Figure 3.19

Verification of licensure: Federation of State Medical Boards

[Date]

To: Disciplinary Inquiries
    Federation of State Medical Boards
    400 Fuller Wise Road, Suite 300
    Euless, TX 76039-3855

Re: *[Reapplicant's full name]*
    Social Security Number:
    Date of birth:
    School:
    Year graduated:
    ECFMG #:

To Whom It May Concern:

Please conduct a disciplinary action search on the above-referenced practitioner. Enclosed with this letter is a copy of a release and immunity statement. This statement constitutes consent to this inquiry and to your response, and releases from liability any individual who provides the requested information.

Please send the results to:

[Name of hospital]
[Hospital contact name and title]
[Address]

Thank you for your kind attention to this matter.

Sincerely,

[Manager, credentialing services]
Enclosures

Figure 3.20

Verification of state controlled substance registration

[Date]

Re: [Name of reapplicant]

To Whom It May Concern:

The above-referenced practitioner has applied for reappointment and continuation of clinical privileges at [Hospital name].

Please verify this practitioner's controlled substance registration status in your state. We would appreciate it if you would provide the information requested on the attachment (if pertinent to this practitioner). After completing the attachment, please return it to us in the enclosed envelope. Also enclosed with this letter is a copy of a release and immunity statement. This statement constitutes consent to this inquiry and to your response, and releases from liability any individual who provides the requested information.

We appreciate your prompt and full reply.

Sincerely,

[Manager, credentialing services]
Enclosures

Figure 3.21

Verification of state controlled substance registration questionnaire

Controlled substance number: _____

Date issued: _____ Date expires: _____

If not yet issued, indicate date applied:_____

Has your agency ever initiated or taken any action during the time period under review, or is any action currently pending to revoke, suspend, limit, modify, terminate, relinquish, restrict or make probationary, or otherwise investigate or challenge any matters involving the applicant's controlled substance registration?
❑ Yes   ❑ No

If yes, please provide details: _____
_____
_____
_____
_____

List all schedules of drugs the applicant is registered to prescribe: _____
_____
_____
_____
_____

Verified and completed by: _____

Name (type or print):_____ Title: _____

Signature: _____ Date: _____

Return to: *[Hospital name]*
      Attn: *[Manager, credentialing services]*
      [Address]

Figure 3.22 — Verification of professional liability insurance

[Date]
Request #:

Re:
Policy #:
Coverage period:

To Whom It May Concern:

The above-named practitioner has applied for reappointment to our medical staff and for continuation of clinical privileges. In evaluating this reapplicant, we must investigate his or her professional liability coverage experience during the most recent appointment period.

Please complete the enclosed questionnaire and return it in the enclosed envelope. Your prompt and full reply will be appreciated. Also enclosed is a copy of a signed release and immunity statement. This statement constitutes consent to this inquiry and to your response and releases from liability any individual who provides the requested information.

Sincerely,

[Manager, credentialing services]
Enclosures

Figure 3.23

Professional liability insurance and experience questionnaire

[Date]

Re: [Full name of practitioner]
Carrier: _____
Policy #: _____
Policy period: _____

1. We provide(d) professional liability insurance under the policy referenced for the above-named
   practitioner.   ❑ Yes   ❑ No

   If yes, please complete questions 2, 3, and 4 below.

2. a. Type of insurance: _____
      Claims made: _____
      Occurrence: _____

   b. Coverage period: _____
                          from (Mo/Day/Yr)   to (Mo/Day/Yr)

   c. Coverage amounts: _____ / _____

3. Have you ever cancelled or not renewed this practitioner's insurance, or imposed a specific surcharge
   based on the individual's experience?   ❑ Yes   ❑ No

   If yes, when and for what reasons? _____
   _____
   _____

4. Have there ever been or are there currently pending any challenges, claims, settlements, or judgments
   against this practitioner?   ❑ Yes   ❑ No

   If yes, please summarize on a separate sheet of paper and attach it to this questionnaire.

5. Have any specific procedures been excluded from this practitioner's coverage?
                                                                        ❑ Yes   ❑ No

   If yes, please list the procedures: _____
   _____
   _____

Completed by (print): _____

_____
Signature   Title   Date

Figure 3.24 — Verification of specialty board certification

[Date]

Executive Director
[Name of organization/board]

[Practitioner's full name (including any other names used)]
Specialty:
Social security number:
Date of birth:
Year certified:

To Whom It May Concern:

The above-mentioned practitioner has applied for reappointment to the *[Hospital name]* medical staff and for continuation of clinical privileges.

In evaluating the application, we must verify certification status. We would appreciate your completing the attached statement or providing the equivalent information on your own form and returning it to us in the enclosed envelope. Your prompt and full reply will be appreciated.

Also enclosed is a copy of a signed release and immunity statement. This statement constitutes consent to this inquiry and to your response, and releases from liability any individual who provides this information.

Sincerely,

[Manager, credentialing services]
Enclosures

Figure 3.25 Verification of specialty board certification status

[Date]

Specialty:
Specialty board:

Overall area and any special certificates held and the date certified in each.

Area certified in: _____

Year certified: _____

Valid until: _____

Currently in the certification examination process?   ❑ Yes   ❑ No

Date entered process: _____
Date by which process must be completed: _____
Requirements remaining: _____
_____

Failed examination during time period under review?   ❑ Yes   ❑ No

If yes, when? _____ Oral _____ Written _____

Currently is in the process of seeking recertification?   ❑ Yes   ❑ No   ❑ N/A

Verified and completed by: _____

Name (type or print): _____ Title: _____

Signature: _____ Date: _____

Return to: [Hospital name]
        Attn: [Manager, credentialing services]
        [Address]

Figure 3.26

Letter for verification of additional school or training

[Date]

Office of the Dean or Registrar

Re: *[Reapplicant's name]*
 Social security number:
 Date of birth:
 Dates attended:

Dear Sir/Madam:

The above-named practitioner has applied for reappointment to the medical staff of *[Hospital name]*. The reapplication indicates that he/she attended and/or graduated from your school during the period indicated above. As part of our reappointment process, we must verify this information.

Please assist us by completing the information on the following page and returning it to us in the enclosed envelope. Also enclosed is a copy of a signed release and immunity statement. This statement constitutes consent to this inquiry and your response, and releases from liability any individual who provides the requested information. Your prompt reply will be appreciated.

Sincerely,

[Manager, credentialing services]
Enclosures

Figure 3.27

Verification of attendance at/or graduation from professional school

[Date]
[School name]
[City], [State] [County]

Dates attended: _____
from (Mo/Yr)   through (Mo/Yr)

Degree awarded: _____ Date: _____
(Mo/Yr)

Cumulative GPA: _____

If a degree was not awarded and the individual is no longer in the program, please explain the circumstances surrounding or give the reason for the individual's departure:

Verified and completed by: _____

Name (type or print): _____ Title: _____

Signature: _____ Date: _____

Return to: [Hospital name]
      Attn: [Manager, credentialing services]
      [Address]

Figure 3.28 — Verification of additional training

[Date]

Re: *[Reapplicant's name]*
    Specialty:
    Dates:

Dear Sir/Madam:

The above-named individual has applied for reappointment to the medical staff of *[Hospital name]* for continuation of clinical privileges. His/her reapplication states that the above training took place at your institution.

Would you please verify this information by completing the questions and rating scale on the following page? If you do not have adequate knowledge to answer a particular question or to provide a rating, please indicate "No Information." Enclosed is a copy of a release and immunity statement signed by the practitioner consenting to this inquiry and your response. It releases from liability any individual who provides the requested information. Your full and prompt reply is appreciated.

Thank you for your assistance.

Sincerely,

[Manger, Credentialing Services]
Enclosures

Figure 3.29 — **Verification of training questionnaire**

[Date]

If you answer "no" or "none" to questions 1, 2, or 3, please provide an explanation on a separate sheet.

1. a. Was the practitioner at your institution in the indicated program for the
stated period of time? ❑ Yes ❑ No

   b. Was the program accredited at the time the practitioner participated in it? ❑ Yes ❑ No

   c. Did he/she successfully complete the program? ❑ Yes ❑ No

2. If a residency program, did the practitioner attain the status of chief resident? ❑ Yes ❑ No

   If yes, please indicate the term as chief resident.

3. Of the privileges/services requested on the attached form, for which is the
practitioner qualified by the training and/or experience received in the above
program and by his/her performance in the program?

If you answer "Yes" to any of questions 4 through 11, please provide an explanation on a separate sheet.

4. Was the practitioner ever subject to or considered for disciplinary action? ❑ Yes ❑ No

5. Did the practitioner ever attempt procedures beyond his/her skill or
assigned training protocols? ❑ Yes ❑ No

6. Was the practitioner's status and/or authority to provide services ever revoked,
suspended, reduced, restricted, not renewed or was he/she placed on
probationary status or reprimanded at any time? ❑ Yes ❑ No

7. Were proceedings ever initiated that could have led to any of
the actions in #6? ❑ Yes ❑ No

8. Did the practitioner ever voluntarily terminate his/her status in the
program or any particular privileges/services, or restrict the same,
in lieu of formal action or to avoid an investigation? ❑ Yes ❑ No

---

Figure 3.29 | **Verification of training questionnaire (cont.)**

Professional knowledge, skills, and attitude

9. Please review the attached delineation of privileges/services form(s) and refer to the form as appropriate in completing the following chart below. If you do not have adequate knowledge to answer a particular question, please indicate "No Information."

Please rate the following:
Basic medical/clinical knowledge
a. Knowledge in specialty
b. Technical skills
c. Clinical judgment
d. Availability and thoroughness in caring for patients
e. Appropriate use of consultants in timely manner
f. Quality/appropriateness of care provided
g. Appropriateness of resource use
    (admissions, procedures, tests, therapies, etc.)
h. Clarity and completeness of medical record content
i. Medical record timeliness
j. Legibility of records
k. Participation in committees, officership/leadership
l. Verbal and written fluency in English
m. Rapport with patients
n. Ability to work with others

10. Please use this section for any additional comments, information, or recommendations that may be relevant to our decision to renew the practitioner's appointment/affiliation and clinical privileges/services.

_____

_____

11. My recommendation concerning this practitioner's application for reappointment/affiliation is as follows:
    ❏ Recommended   ❏ Recommended with conditions   ❏ Not recommended

12. My recommendation concerning the specific clinical privileges/services requested is as follows:
    ❏ Would recommend for all requested
    ❏ Would limit certain privileges/services
    ❏ Would not recommend certain privileges/services
    ❏ Would not recommend for any privileges/services

Completed by: _____

Name (type or print): _____ Title: _____

Signature: _____ Date: _____

Information provided based on the following (check all that apply):
❏ Direct knowledge   ❏ File record   ❏ Direct knowledge in part/file record in part

Return to: *[Hospital name]*
            Attn: *[Manager, credentialing services]*
            [Address]

Figure 3.30

Letter to appointee requesting assistance obtaining information for reappointment application

Dear Dr. *[Practitioner name]*:

During the processing of your request for reappointment to our medical staff, we sent the attached letter(s) and questionnaire(s) to the *[Chief executive officer/applicable department chair(s)/medical records director]* of *[Hospital name]*. To date, we have not received a reply and are therefore unable to forward your application for reappointment to our credentials committee.

With this letter I am requesting your assistance in this matter. I have enclosed a second copy of the questionnaire(s) to *[Hospital name]*. Please have the proper representative(s) of the aforementioned Hospital return the questionnaire(s) and associated information to my attention as soon as possible. Once we have received this information, it will be submitted to the credentials committee with your application for reappointment.

If we do not receive the information requested above within 15 days of the date of this letter, we will be unable to process your application for reappointment and your appointment at our hospital will expire. We appreciate your cooperation in this matter and look forward to your continued affiliation with our hospital.

Sincerely,

[Chief executive officer]
Enclosure

Figure 3.31

Reappointment questionnaire to be completed by the chief executive officer of another practice affiliation

Dr. *[Practitioner name]* is currently reapplying for appointment to the medical staff of this Hospital. Please verify the following information.

1. Dr. *[Practitioner name]* holds _____ category
   status in your medical staff. ❑ Yes ❑ No

2. Dr. *[Practitioner name]* has clinical privileges in the department of
   _____. ❑ Yes ❑ No

3. Dr. *[Practitioner name]*'s appointment and/or clinical privileges have not been
   reduced, suspended, or diminished in any way either through voluntary or
   involuntary means. ❑ Yes ❑ No

4. In general, Dr. *[Practitioner name]* relates to other professionals and hospital
   employees in a manner that is conducive to good hospital/staff patient
   relations. ❑ Yes ❑ No

5. Please provide this hospital with your personal recommendation concerning Dr. *[Practitioner name]*'s
   request for reappointment and clinical privileges for the next two years.

   ❑ Recommend for reappointment and clinical privileges
   ❑ Cannot recommend for reappointment and/or clinical privileges
   ❑ I am unable to formulate a recommendation for the following reasons: _____
   _____

   ❑ Other (please specify): _____

_____   _____
Chief executive officer's signature   Name of organization

Figure 3.32

Reappointment questionnaire to be completed by the applicable department chair of another hospital affiliation

Note: *A copy of the appointee's current clinical privileges should accompany this questionnaire.*

Re: *[Practitioner name]*   Date of birth: _____

Specialty: _____

The above-referenced practitioner is currently reapplying for appointment to the medical staff of this hospital. We would appreciate your help in providing the following information.

1. Please rate the following:

	Satisfactory	Unsatisfactory	Don't know
Clinical knowledge	❑	❑	❑
Clinical competence	❑	❑	❑
Emotional stability*	❑	❑	❑
Work habits	❑	❑	❑
Participation in staff/committee activities	❑	❑	❑
Relationship with patients	❑	❑	❑
Relationship with peers	❑	❑	❑
Relationship with hospital staff	❑	❑	❑
Professional attitude	❑	❑	❑
Character	❑	❑	❑
Ability to work with others	❑	❑	❑

2. Dr. *[Practitioner name]* was on the medical records suspension list *[number]* times in the past 12 months.

Summary recommendations

❑ I recommend without reservation for appointment with all requested privileges.

❑ I recommend with reservation as noted on the attached privileges list.

❑ I do not recommend this applicant.

❑ I cannot comment on the clinical competence of the individual referenced above.

_____   _____
Department chair's signature   Name of organization

_____
Date

All organizations must comply with the Americans with Disabilities Act.

Figure 3.33 — Letter requesting information from other practice affiliations

Re: *[Practitioner name]*
Date of birth: _____
Period of requested information: _____

Dear *[insert name of CEO/department chair/medical records director]*:

The purpose of this letter is to request your assistance as we process a request for reappointment from the above-referenced practitioner on our medical staff. Enclosed is a copy of a signed release and immunity statement, consenting to this inquiry and your response and releasing from liability any individual who provides the requested information.

This applicant indicates that he/she is currently a member in good standing of your medical staff. Because he/she has had relatively little clinical activity at our hospital, we must rely on information provided by you.

Please understand that we do not need, nor will we use, this information for competitive reasons. The information you provide will be used solely for the processing of his/her request for reappointment, as we attempt to determine his/her current clinical competence in the area of his/her requested privileges.

The attached questionnaire outlines the information that our credentials committee would like. If this information is costly to provide, please feel free to submit an invoice with your completed questionnaire.

Thank you very much for assisting us in this issue.

Sincerely,

Chief executive officer
Enclosure

Figure 3.34 **Reappointment questionnaire to be completed by the medical records director of other hospital or practice affiliation**

Note: If this questionnaire is to be sent without an accompanying letter, a copy of the medical staff member's signed release and immunity statement must be enclosed.

Re: *[Practitioner name]*   Date of birth: _____

Specialty: _____

Period of requested information: From __/___/__ to __/___/___

Dr. *[Practitioner name]* is currently reapplying for appointment to the medical staff of this hospital. He states that he holds medical staff membership and clinical privileges at your facility. We ask that you provide the following information as applicable to his practice at your facility.

1. Number of admissions _____
2. Number of surgeries _____
3. Number of invasive procedures _____
4. Number of consults _____
5. Number of patients attended in the critical care unit _____
6. Number of times on medical records suspension _____
7. Average length of patient stay _____
8. Number of mortalities _____
9. If you have a physician summary or profile report available that reflects the number and type of patients treated by this physician, that report alone will suffice, in lieu of the previously requested information. Please attach the report if you so desire.

Special note: All information supplied above must be authenticated by the medical records director and his/her signature must appear at the bottom of this form.

I have provided this information for use in the credentialing process at *[Hospital name]*. To the best of my knowledge, this information accurately reflects this physician's clinical activity at our hospital during the above-referenced time period.

_____   _____
Signature, Medical records director   Name of hospital

_____
Date

Figure 3.35

Department chair reappointment recommendation

Re: Appointee *[Practitioner name]*   Reappointment expiration date: _____

In my professional opinion, Dr. *[Practitioner name]* is qualified for reappointment to this hospital's medical staff with continued clinical privileges as follows:

Staff category

❏ Active

❏ Associate

❏ Honorary

Department affiliation

❏ Surgery

❏ Medicine

❏ Other _____

This finding is based upon the following appraisals:

	Satisfactory	Needs improvement	Unsatisfactory
Level of activity	❏	❏	❏
Clinical competence	❏	❏	❏
Technical skill/judgment	❏	❏	❏
Professional performance based on the results of QA/I activity	❏	❏	❏
Ability to relate well with peers	❏	❏	❏
Ability to relate well with staff	❏	❏	❏
Ability to relate well with patients	❏	❏	❏
Adherence to medical staff bylaws	❏	❏	❏
Health status*	❏	❏	❏

In addition, I recommend that Dr. *[Practitioner name]* be granted privileges as shown on the attached clinical privilege request form.

Comment(s) _____

_____

_____

Department chair's signature   Date

*All organizations must abide by the Americans with Disabilities Act.

Figure 3.36

Reappointment profile/summary

Name _____ Time frame of review _____

Department affiliation _____ Staff category _____

Clinical privileges/specialty _____

Clinical activity data

_____ # of admissions   _____ # of consults performed

_____ # of surgical procedures   _____ # of consults ordered

_____ # of invasive procedures   _____ # of emergency room contacts

Membership Information

	Year 2000	Year 2001
Meeting attendance (50%)	___(#)___/___%	___(#)___/___%
Medical staff meetings	___(#)___/___%	___(#)___/___%
Committee meetings (if any)	___(#)___/___%	___(#)___/___%
Department meetings	___(#)___/___%	___(#)___/___%

Evidence of CME on file   ❑ Yes   ❑ No   # of hours _____   *(40 hours CME category 1 required)*

Number of times on medical records suspension _____

Number of delinquent records _____

Reappointment dues paid (if required)   ❑ Yes   ❑ No

License and DEA number verified   ❑ Yes   ❑ No

National Practitioner Data Bank report received   ❑ Yes   ❑ No

Professional liability insurance verified   ❑ Yes   ❑ No

Any OIG or state sanctions   ❑ Yes*   ❑ No

Any known felony criminal actions   ❑ Yes*   ❑ No

Any patient/staff complaints   ❑ Yes*   ❑ No

*Comments

_____

_____

Figure 3.36

Reappointment profile/summary (cont.)

Clinical profile

Gross data

Overall mortality rate _____

Average length of stay _____

Number of autopsies ordered _____

Disciplinary action (previous two years) _____

Number of documented patient/staff/complaints _____

Number of malpractice claims filed _____

Note: *Attach the physician profile/report to this form, along with a summary of pertinent quality assurance/improvement data.*

Gynecology monitoring   Number of charts reviewed _____

Indicator number	1	2	3	4	5	6	7	8	9	10	11	12	13	14	15	16
Number of variations																
Departmental average																

Medical monitoring   Number of charts reviewed _____

Indicator number	1	2	3	4	5	6	7	8	9	10	11	12	13	14	15	16
Number of variations																
Departmental average																

Pediatric monitoring   Number of charts reviewed _____

Indicator number	1	2	3	4	5	6	7	8	9	10	11	12	13	14	15	16
Number of variations																
Departmental average																

Surgical monitoring   Number of charts reviewed _____

Indicator number	1	2	3	4	5	6	7	8	9	10	11	12	13	14	15	16
Number of variations																
Departmental average																

Figure 3.36

Reappointment profile/summary (cont.)

(Note presence or absence of significant problems identified through review activity.)

Surgical case review _____

Antibiotic and drug use review _____

Blood use review _____

Special care unit care review

Mortality review _____

Utilization review _____

Medical records review _____

Departmental review _____

Figure 3.37 | Monitoring form

This form and the following monitoring indicators may be used to collect the data that is required for reappointment activity summaries. Alternatively, hospitals might use their existing quality assurance/improvement program to identify specific quality-of-care indicators that department chairs would like reported for each physician.

Medical record number _____

Admitting diagnosis _____

Attending physician number _____

Final diagnosis _____

Patient age/sex _____

Length of stay _____

Indicators

_____

_____

_____

Comments

_____

_____

_____

_____

_____

Figure 3.38 | **Sample monitoring indicators**

Gynecology

1. GYN patients with transfusions
2. Preoperative and postoperative diagnoses do not agree
3. Postoperative stay over seven days
4. Malignancy
5. Patient received more than two antibiotics concurrently
6. Readmission within one month of discharge
7. Complications: Morbidity (temperature > 100.4 for two consecutive days)
8. Patient returned to the operating room this admission
9. Unplanned removal or repair of an organ or part of an organ during operative procedure
10. Mortality

Medical

1. Justification for admission
2. Readmission within four weeks
3. Diagnosis made within 72 hours
4. Return to ICU
5. Antibiotic with no culture and sensitivity
6. More than two antibiotics at the same time
7. Transfusion
8. Length of stay > 10 days
9. Transfer to another hospital
10. Mortality

Pediatric

1. Readmissions for same condition within one year before this admission
2. Mortality
3. Transfusions
4. Nonspecific diagnosis (i.e., symptoms only) at discharge

Figure 3.38 **Sample monitoring indicators (cont.)**

5. Temperature > 103 oral at least once daily for more than 96 hours

6. Febrile (i.e., > 100 oral; >100 rectal) within 24 hours before discharge

7. Length of stay > five days

8. Transfer to another hospital

9. Antibiotics without culture and sensitivity

Note: Pediatric monitoring includes all nonsurgical patients less than 15 years of age and those 15 to 18 years of age under the care of pediatricians.

Surgical

1. Readmission to this hospital within six months for complications or because of incomplete management of problem treated on previous admission

2. Patient transferred from general care to special care or isolation unit (e.g., ICU, CCU, isolation)

3. Patient transferred to another acute care facility

4. Patient returned to operating room on this admission

5. Patient operated on for repair of laceration, perforation, tear, or puncture of an organ subsequent to procedure or unplanned removal of an organ during a procedure

6. Acute myocardial infarction and surgical procedure on same admission

7. Wound infection or temperature > 101 lasting a full day before and/or on day of discharge

8. Neurological deficit (not present at admission or before surgery) on last full day before and/or on day of discharge

9. Mortality

10. Cardiac or respiratory arrest

11. Transfusions

12. Discrepancy between final and pathological diagnoses

Figure 3.39

Reappraisal/Reappointment documentation checklist

The information listed below must be in each medical staff appointee's reappointment file in order for the file to be complete.

Re: *[Practitioner name]*
Assigned department: _____

	Yes	No
Request for reappointment and clinical privileges—completed reappointment information form, including requested		
• clinical privileges and information regarding clinical privileges	❑	❑
• health status*	❑	❑
• sanctions	❑	❑
• licensure status	❑	❑
• evidence of professional liability coverage and malpractice history	❑	❑
• evidence of continuing medical education	❑	❑
• National Practitioner Data Bank report	❑	❑
• Federation of State Medical Board report	❑	❑
• Other hospital affiliation information	❑	❑
• Any OIG or state sanction	❑	❑
• Criminal background check, if applicable	❑	❑
Clinical information pertaining to performance		
• summary of clinical activity including number and types of patients treated	❑	❑
• information demonstrating current clinical competence	❑	❑
• review of department and committee minutes	❑	❑
• clinical data demonstrating outcome of clinical activity	❑	❑
Evidence that the above information was reviewed by the		
• department chair	❑	❑
• credentials committee	❑	❑
• medical executive committee	❑	❑
• governing board	❑	❑
Evidence that the recommendation was submitted to the governing board by the MEC	❑	❑

Compiled by: _____
Date: _____ Title: _____

*All organizations must abide by the Americans with Disabilities Act.

Figure 3.40

Malpractice review policy

Policy statement:

There will be a thorough review of malpractice cases during the credentialing process for initial and reappointment applicants.

Procedure and criteria for review:

1. Malpractice claims are identified by the credentialing specialist upon receipt and application processing, or by other members of the medical staff, credentials committee, or administration.

2. For initial applications, information related to malpractice is flagged and reviewed by the appropriate department chair and vice president of medical affairs (VPMA) during initial screening.

3. For reappointment applications, information related to malpractice is flagged and reviewed by the appropriate department chair during the privilege approval/file review-credentialing phase.

4. All reported malpractice claims (open or closed) are reviewed by the credentials committee chair prior to submission to the credentials committee.

5. The department chairs, credentials committee chair, and/or VPMA determine and convey to the credentialing specialist the adequacy of information provided and the need for further information if indicated.

6. The credentialing specialist will make available in the credentials committee agenda packet (said packet to be duly and clearly marked "confidential" and "to be opened by addressee only") the following information regarding malpractice cases:

   a. Nature of allegation/severity of claim/patient outcome
   b. Naming of practitioner (primary defendant, co-defendant, etc.)
   c. Date of act/omission/occurrence, and date case closed
   d. Disposition of case
   e. Amount of settlement, if any
   f. Practitioner statement

The above lettered information will be provided for all closed claims upon initial application, and for claims closed during the previous two-year-period for reappointment applications. Additionally, open

---

Figure 3.40 | **Malpractice review policy (cont.)**

claims for both initial and reappointment applicants will be provided when the information is deemed pertinent by the department chair/credentials chair to identify trends related to the provision of adequate standard of patient care.

7. The credentials committee will review malpractice information noting trends/significant aspects of each case as one measurement to assess competency, and referring to the *Midwest Medical Insurance Company's "Most Prevalent Misadventures per Specialty"* information.

8. If trends/patterns are identified, the applicant will be invited to participate in an interview with the VPMA, medical staff president, credentials chair, department chair, like specialty/clinical director, and others as indicated (chief executive office, medical staff office, legal counsel, etc.) to determine whether specific outcome monitors should be established and reported to the credentials committee and department chair.

9. In the event the credentials committee is unable to make a determination based on a comprehensive review of all applicant information, outside consultation will be sought.

10. The credentials committee will not recommend membership or privilege denial based solely upon the number of claims, or a claims threshold criteria, but may deny membership or privileges based upon a complete review of credentialing information required and available for review.

11. Recommended action will be forwarded with findings to the medical executive committee, having authority to convey said recommended action approval or revised recommended action to the credentials committee, who in turn may communicate the medical executive committee determination to the applicant for response.

12. In the event adverse action is recommended, the applicant will be advised of his/her right to fair hearing and appellate review procedures as described in the medical staff bylaws.

13. When applicant acceptance of recommended action, or resolution via the fair hearing and appellate review process occurs, the recommendation will be forwarded to the board of trustees for final approval.

Source: Children's Hospital, Omaha, NE. Reprinted with permission.

| Figure 3.41 | Policy regarding exchange of credentialing, performance improvement, and peer review information |

I. Purpose

Components (hospitals, managed care organizations, surgicenters, and ambulatory facilities, etc.) of this corporation wish to share information that is reasonably related to the qualifications, competency, ability, professional ethics, and conduct of the practitioners providing patient care within the components.

The corporation believes that by sharing this information, it can

- improve the quality of care
- improve the quality of available quality improvement data by increasing the size of the data pool
- facilitate the development of consistency in the application of professional standards and quality assessment throughout the system
- reduce duplication of administrative procedures, professional peer reviews, and investigations
- reduce the cost of the credentialing process

Because the corporation's board of directors/trustees is responsible for the overall management of the corporation, it has adopted this policy to provide for the exchange of credentialing information within the corporation and its various components.

II. Policy

"Credentialing information," as defined below, is confidential and privileged and should be managed appropriately. The credentialing information outlined below may be exchanged within the components and related organizations of this corporation in accordance with this policy.

"Credentialing information" includes all information, applications, references, data, and reports that relate to the qualifications, competency, ability to practice, professional ethics, or conduct of a medical/professional staff applicant or member. It includes, but is not limited to, the following:

1. Initial application and all supporting materials of all medical/professional staff applicants.

2. Application for reappointment to, or renewal of, membership on the medical/professional staff and all supporting materials for the medical/professional staff, including, but not limited to, the following:

    - Quality assessment and improvement information

Figure 3.41 | **Policy regarding exchange of credentialing, performance improvement, and peer review information (cont.)**

- Stipulations or conditions of the board of medical practice (examiners) or other appropriate licensing agency
- Restrictions, conditions, or limitations established by the corporation
- Reports of peer review committees, proctors, monitors, or consultants
- Administrative suspensions, including medical records suspensions
- Other information or data believed to be supportive of quality patient care or the efficient operation of the organization

3. Information on the status (requested, granted, or denied) of an applicant's privileges, membership, or panel appointment at any component of a corporation.

4. Any reports or correspondence regarding a medical/professional staff applicant or member that were sent to a state licensing agency (e.g., the board of medical practice or board of nursing), the National Practitioner Data Bank, the peer review organization authorized by Medicare, or any other governmental agency that receives such reports.

5. Reports, assessments, incident reports, and other information gathered under peer review or by the administration or staff of the corporation. The corporation may exchange this information when it reasonably related to the quality of care, efficient delivery of care, or the competency of a practitioner. The corporation may also share incident reports regarding disruptive and inappropriate behavior if a peer review committee believes that such conduct or pattern of conduct interferes with the delivery of patient care, poses a threat to the safety of patients or staff members, or creates a hostile working environment.

6. Information regarding necessary accommodations or restrictions made to the privileges, duties, or work performed by a medical/professional staff member due to any health condition or disability. Such information is confidential, and only those individuals and committees responsible for supervising and managing the medical/professional staff shall have access to it.

III. Conditions for exchange of credentialing information

A. Authorization by practitioner. The corporation may exchange credentialing information in accordance with this policy once it receives a release signed by the medical/professional staff applicant or member. The release will remain valid unless and until it is revoked by the applicant or member in

---

Figure 3.41 | **Policy regarding exchange of credentialing, performance improvement, and peer review information (cont.)**

---

writing. Each medical/professional staff applicant or member must authorize the release of credentialing information as a condition of consideration of his or her application for membership, appointment, reappointment, or renewal.

B. **Exchange of credentialing information.** The appropriate credentialing and/or membership committee of the corporation (or their designees) shall exchange credentialing information to assess professional qualifications and grant membership or privileges in order to improve the quality of patient care, or for some other appropriate reason. Each committee must agree to maintain confidentiality of the credentialing information and to restrict the use of such information to the purposes set forth in state statutes.

C. **Patient-specific information.** The corporation must remove all identifying information before exchanging credentialing information that relates to the care of, treatment of, or relationship with a specific patient, unless otherwise authorized in writing by the patient or corporation. When appropriate and practical, the corporation shall exchange patient data in the form of aggregate data or summaries.

D. **Minutes/discussion of peer review committees.** The corporation may exchange minutes or actions of any peer review committee only if such materials are reviewed and edited to remove the following.

- Patient identification (if any)
- The identities of individuals participating in or providing information to the committee
- All comments, quotations, or discussions made by the participants during the review

E. **Required statements.** All credentialing information exchanged in accordance with this policy shall include the label "confidential credentialing information," accompanied by the following statement:

The attached credentialing information is confidential health care review data under state statutes. Disclosure of all or any part of the attached information is not subject to discovery by subpoena or otherwise, nor may it be introduced into evidence in any administrative or judicial proceeding except as required or permitted by law. The recipient is responsible for maintaining the confidentiality of the attached information.

Figure 3.41 | **Policy regarding exchange of credentialing, performance improvement, and peer review information (cont.)**

F. **Security and confidentiality.** The corporation is responsible for taking adequate measures to protect the privileged and confidential nature of the credentialing information exchanged in accordance with this policy. The corporation providing credentialing information in accordance with this policy is entitled to rely on the receiving corporation to provide adequate security for the information and to use such information only as authorized under this policy.

G. **Coordination with risk management.** The corporation is responsible for coordinating the exchange of information under this policy with the risk manager or other personnel responsible for reviewing and assessing potential liability for the corporation.

IV. Scope of policy

A. **Entity specifying determinations.** The corporation is responsible for and will have the authority to make any determinations regarding membership or privileges at the corporation. Nothing in this policy is intended to limit the authority of the corporation to take such actions as they deem appropriate regarding the qualifications, competency, or ability to practice of any medical/professional staff applicant or member.

B. **Events triggering exchange of information.** The exchange of credentialing information will take place in accordance with this policy upon the following events:

  • The request of the corporation's membership committee and/or credentials committee
  • The determination of the corporation's membership committee and/or credentials committee that it knows of information that it believes should be exchanged to advance the purposes of this policy or improve patient care
  • An individual's initial application for membership or privileges, or application for reappointment or renewal to the corporation's medical/professional staff

Note: This policy can easily be modified for use by managed care organizations and corporations wishing to exchange or share applicable information.

Source: The Top Twenty-Five Medical Staff Policies and Procedures, Second Edition, *copyright 2002 HCPro, Inc., Marblehead, MA.*

Figure 3.42

Notification to practitioner of favorable reappointment

Note: Send by certified mail, return receipt requested, or by courier/messenger with signed acknowledgement of receipt.

[Date]

Dear *[Reapplicant's name]*:

On behalf of the Board of *[directors/trustees]*, it is my pleasure to inform you that your appointment to the medical staff of *[insert hospital name]* has been renewed for the following staff category and clinical department/sections.

Category: *[active, courtesy, consulting, as applicable]*

Department: *[medicine, surgery, anesthesia, as applicable]*

Section: *[cardiology, general surgery]*

Your clinical privilege requests have been approved and are granted as specified on the enclosed copy of the clinical privilege forms.

This appointment and the clinical privileges are effective from *[date of board action]* until *[date two years from board action]* unless changed or resigned pursuant to the appropriate sections of the medical staff bylaws and related documents.

Thank you for your past support of *[Hospital name]*. We look forward to your continued support and participation in medical staff activities.

Sincerely,

[Chief executive officer]
cc: *[Department chair]*
Enclosure

Figure 3.43

Notification of adverse reappointment determination

[Date]

Dear [Reapplicant's name]:

With utmost regret I inform you that the medical executive committee has decided to recommend to the board of *[trustees/directors]* the denial of your request for reappointment to the medical staff of *[hospital name]* and your continuation of clinical privileges. The reasons for the medical executive committee's decision are as follows:

[Summarize recommendation/action not to reappoint, and/or deny or restrict requested clinical privileges.]

You may request a formal hearing by submitting your request in writing to my attention, delivered in person or by certified mail within 30 calendar days of receipt of this letter.

Failure to request a formal hearing within that time period and in the manner specified will be deemed a waiver of your right to a hearing and to any appellate review to which you might have been entitled and will indicate your acceptance of the action recommended without further recourse.

Upon receipt of a timely request for a hearing, you will be notified at least 30 calendar days in advance of the date, time, and place of the hearing. Please refer to the copy of the fair hearing plan enclosed for a full description of our hearing and appellate review process.

Further, please also note that the medical executive committee's action, if endorsed by the board of *[trustees/directors]*, may be reported to the state medical board and to the National Practitioner Data Bank, as required by law. You will be provided with a copy of any report that is filed, and given an opportunity to submit a rebuttal or further information.

Sincerely,

[Chief of staff]
Enclosure

Figure 3.44

Notification to hospital/medical staff departments of reappointments

[Date]

To: Department chairs
 Section chiefs

From: Dr. *[name]*, chief of staff/medical staff president
Re: Reappointments to the medical staff

Effective *[date of board action]*, the following practitioners have been reappointed to the medical staff with the category and department/section affiliations shown below:

Practitioner section	Category	Department
_____	_____	_____
_____	_____	_____
_____	_____	_____
_____	_____	_____
_____	_____	_____
_____	_____	_____
_____	_____	_____

A copy of the clinical privileges granted to each of the above practitioners who is a member or has been granted privileges in your department or section is attached for your records.

cc: *[appropriate hospital department(s) on a need-to-know basis (e.g., medical records, operating suite, admitting, emergency department, etc.)]*

Enclosure

Chapter 4

Clinical

Privileges

Clinical Privileges

The Joint Commission on Accreditation of Healthcare Organization's (JCAHO) reappointment standards require hospitals to follow a process that is very similar to the one followed when processing an applicant's request for initial appointment. Reappointment standards require medical staff services professionals to gather and verify credentials information, appropriate groups and individuals to review the complete credentials file, and the governing board to make a final decision regarding reappointment and clinical privileges based on the result of those reviews.

Clinical privilege delineation—the process a hospital follows to determine the procedures each medical staff appointee may perform and the conditions he or she can treat—is an important step in the reappointment process and must be done fairly and consistently. This step is critical to ensuring that the hospital reappoints only those physicians who maintain the competency to perform requested privileges.

Analyzing a practitioner's education, training, and experience, and matching this information with the procedures he or she wishes to perform and conditions he or she seeks to treat can be one of the greatest challenges faced by a credentials committee and hospital board during the reappointment process.

Physicians applying for reappointment must specify requested modifications to his or her clinical privileges at least 60 days prior to the expiration of his or her medical staff appointment. The practitioner must also provide evidence of his or her current clinical competence in the privileges re-quested. Provide the practitioner with a new request for clinical privileges and a list of his or her current clinical privileges. The physician must then complete the new privilege request form by reviewing that list and making necessary changes.

Industry changes

The traditional strategies hospitals used to delineate privileges are outdated because of the progress of new technology and the proliferation of new subspecialty areas. The delineation of clinical privileges—with the ultimate goal of ensuring patient quality—has become increasingly more complex as organizations attempt to comply with JCAHO requirements. The process must also minimize a hospital's legal risk, eliminate internal medical staff conflicts, and save valuable time.

In light of these factors, many hospitals and their medical staff leaders have found it daunting to create a process for privilege delineation that complies with accreditor and federal regulations guiding appointment and reappointment. However, it is apparent that hospitals need a system for effective privilege delineation. This system must be flexible enough to add the new procedures physicians wish to perform and conditions they wish to treat, but also be firm, fair, and consistent.

The following section explains why you need threshold criteria, describes the delineation approaches used in the past, and discusses approaches hospitals currently use. It also describes an effective and clinically realistic approach to matching a physician's education, training, and experience with the privileges granted by a hospital.

Develop threshold criteria

Physicians applying for reappointment may request modifications to their clinical privileges that force the hospital to examine its stance on specific procedures, services, and treatments. To grant privileges to practitioners fairly and consistently, a hospital must first determine the services and technologies it will provide. The organization must then outline the minimum qualifications physicians must possess to request clinical privileges. These qualifications are called "minimum threshold criteria."

Distinguish between the criteria for the delineation of clinical privileges and the criteria for medical staff reappointment. The criteria for medical staff reappointment are the general requirements that all applicants reapplying for medical staff appointment, and all physicians currently practicing in the hospital, must meet. To meet the requirements of the JCAHO, state and federal regulators, and hospital boards, a physician must meet specific criteria before the hospital can appoint and reappoint him or her to the medical staff. Criteria could include the following:

- Current license to practice
- Drug Enforcement Administration registration/number
- Professional liability insurance
- Completion of an accredited residency program
- Ability to work well with others

Criteria for delineation of clinical privileges specify the training, experience, and competence needed by the physician to be eligible for specific clinical privileges. The following regulations and issues make this criterion vital:

- **JCAHO standards**—According to the JCAHO's 2003 *Comprehensive Accreditation Manual for Hospitals*, every hospital should have professional criteria as the basis for granting initial, renewed, or modified clinical privileges. These criteria must pertain to, at the very least, evidence of current licensure, relevant training/experience, current competency, and health status.
- **Risk management concerns**—Hospitals that do not set minimum threshold criteria for requesting privileges put themselves at risk of losing accreditation and expose themselves to legal attacks. A hospital can defend itself against a malpractice or corporate liability suit by providing documentation that states a practitioner is qualified to perform all procedures that he or she carries out at the hospital. In addition, antitrust issues can arise if the hospital's process for granting of privileges appears capricious, or if privileging decisions are not based on predefined criteria.
- **Medical staff politics**—Another important consideration is medical staff politics. If there are no written predefined criteria, physicians may feel privileges are not fairly granted. In the past, this has caused significant turmoil within medical staff organizations.
- **Productivity**—Predefined criteria go a long way toward streamlining credentialing and reappointment processes that have become very complex. If criteria are in place for every procedure performed and condition treated at the hospital, the job of deciding whether a physician's training and experience match requested privileges will be much easier. Remember: Some steps in the process can be delegated to nonclinicians to carry out before the request goes to the credentials committee. Thus, only those applicants who meet minimum standards will appear before the committee for review.

Important considerations

Consider the following when developing threshold criteria:

- Privilege criteria should be clinically specific (as opposed to departmentally specific). For example, a hospital's department of surgery may include a variety of specific surgical subspecialties—for example, orthopedics and plastic surgery—that require their own minimum-threshold criteria.
- The chair of the applicable departments or the chiefs of divisions within those departments must recommend the criteria, which the credentials committee, medical executive committee (MEC), and board must then approve.
- The criteria must be met before a request for clinical privileges is complete.

- The hospital should not process any request for clinical privileges that does not meet the minimum criteria. The hospital should instead notify the applicant that his or her request did not meet the minimum threshold criteria and was, therefore, incomplete. In this case, there would be no denial of privileges, no fair hearing, and no report to the state and National Practitioner Data Bank.

- If the applicant does meet the minimum threshold criteria, then the department chair, the credentials committee, MEC, and governing board use professional references and the results of quality assurance to determine whether requests for clinical privileges should be granted.

Note: Credentials committees interested in refining their privileging criteria may be interested in the information contained in three reports. The first was released by the Institute of Medicine. It is entitled *Interpreting the Volume-Outcome Relationship in the Context of Healthcare Quality: Workshop Summary*. The foreword of the document indicates that the volume-outcome relationship may be used to determine the granting of clinical privileges under certain circumstances.

The second report, *The Association Between Hospital Volume and Survival after Acute Myocardial Infarction in Elderly Patients* appeared in a 1999, Volume 340 *New England Journal of Medicine*. The authors of this study found that hospitals that performed low volumes of cardiac surgeries had 17% higher mortality rates than hospitals that handled high volumes of cardiac surgeries. These results suggest that the link between volume and outcomes is strong.

The third report comes from the December 1996 *Effective Health Care*, published by the NHS Center for Reviews and Dissemination at the University of York (UK). The article was entitled "Hospital Volume and Health Care outcomes: Costs and Patient Access."

As organizations continue to publish new research on this topic, it would benefit credentials committees to establish a mechanism for bringing this research to their attention in a timely manner. The Internet should be a valuable tool in facilitating this task. For example, go to *www.google.com* and conduct a search using the keywords "hospital volumes and health care outcomes."

Various approaches to delineating privileges

Hospitals in the United States currently use several methods to match a physician's education, training, and experience with his or her clinical privileges. The following is a brief description of each approach and its limitations:

- **Privilege lists**—Privilege lists, also called "laundry lists," are detailed checklists itemizing the procedures and conditions that medical staff applicants can specifically request. Such lists are often used for surgical specialties.

The greatest failure of this approach is that privilege lists are not often used with predefined criteria. When physicians apply for privileges, they simply check off the procedures they would like to perform and conditions they would like to treat. However, physicians are not often asked to provide specific documentation of training and experience to show they are qualified for those requested privileges.

Another shortcoming of privilege lists is that they are often not inclusive. Because of this drawback, many hospitals are tempted to write "other" at the bottom of the request form, inviting physicians to write in procedures they want to perform or conditions they wish to treat that are not on the list. Hospitals are faced with requests for privileges for which they have no predefined criteria, or for services they do not provide.

Privilege lists can also be restrictive and inflexible. Physicians have been known to apply for all privileges listed instead of taking the time to check only the procedures for which they want privileges—forcing hospitals to deny the physician's request if he or she does not have the necessary training and experience to perform every procedure or treat every condition on the privilege list.

- **Categorization**—Categories, or levels, of privileges, identify major treatment areas or procedures that are classified by the degree of complexity. Occasionally, categories are based on the physician's level of training and experience level or board certification

The JCAHO requires hospitals that use categorization to delineate clinical privileges to develop well-defined categories. The standards that the applicant must meet should be clearly stated for each category. Unfortunately, most hospitals that use this approach create vague categories that make it difficult to match a physician's training and experience to specific privileges.

Because this approach seems to be more applicable to medical areas than to surgical areas, categorization is widely used to delineate privileges in internal or family medicine.

- **Descriptive**—The descriptive approach allows the applicant to describe, in a narrative format, the privileges he or she is requesting. The practitioner is not required to complete a checklist or use categories, but is instead asked to describe those areas in which he or she possesses clinical competence. For example, an orthopedic surgeon may write that he is able to care for patients of all ages with conditions, illness, and injuries of the musculoskeletal system, excluding Laminectomies.

Very few hospitals use this approach to grant physicians clinical privileges. The descriptive approach is most commonly used to delineate privileges for practitioners other than physicians, such as certified nurse-midwives or alcoholism counselors.

- **Combination**—A combination approach combines various features of the laundry list, categorization, and descriptive approaches. Many hospitals list specific privileges within categories, while others may use categories for basic procedures and create lists for those privileges that do not fit into the categories. Still other organizations use a descriptive approach and list privileges that require further consideration.

- **Delineation by codes**—Some hospitals delineate privileges using ICD-9CM and CPT or DRG codes. These codes define the procedures for the credentials committee, MEC, and governing board that would then write the predefined criteria. Assuming an individual meets the predefined criteria for a particular clinical area, he or she is granted privileges based on the ICD-9-CM, CPT or DRG codes for those procedures.

Applicants are required to separately apply for procedures that require specialized training or experience beyond the predefined criteria. The same is true for privileges for a basic procedures done in an unusual fashion, such as performing surgery with a laser instead of a scalpel.

Individuals who do not meet the predefined criteria in a particular clinical area may qualify for limited privileges by providing evidence that they possess training/experience to perform the requested procedures. For example, a family practitioner could apply for procedures on the basic obstetric list, such as cesarean sections. But he or she must demonstrate, to the satisfaction of the board, that he or she possesses satisfactory credentials to warrant the granting of the privilege to perform cesarean sections.

- **Board certification as baseline**—Another approach is to use board certification as a baseline to grant privileges. The hospital adopts specialty board certification or accepts an application to take a certification examination as the criteria for delineation of privileges. For example, if an applicant has just completed an accredited residency and is not yet board-certified, he or she could be granted clinical privileges on the condition of achieving board certification within a specified period of time. Failure to achieve board certification within that time period results in nonrenewal or termination of privileges, unless the hospital board makes an exception.

- **The core privileging approach**—An effective alternative to the laundry list approach is using predefined criteria with a clinically realistic, well-defined description of "core" privileges for each clinical specialty or subspecialty. Core privileging recognizes that the completion of an approved residency training program, and the applicant's practice experience forms the basis for determining competence.

A successful core privileging system should include the following:

• Predefined criteria for each privilege that outline specific education, training and experience requirements

• Accurate, detailed, comprehensive, and specific descriptions of clinical privileges

• A system designed to avoid denials by clearly stating the minimum education, training, and experience needed to apply for specific clinical privileges

For each specialty area, the medical staff (or an appropriate subcommittee) should determine the core set of clinical activities that an appropriately trained physician should be competent to perform. In addition to defining the core set, the medical staff should determine the special requests that require a separate application. Such special requests usually reflect new advances in technology, volume-sensitive privileges, and issues that cross specialty lines.

Figures 4.1–4.7 on pp. 118–130 provide policies, procedures, and forms that your hospital can use to incorporate the core privilege approach in its privileging practices. For more in-depth detail and discussion of how to develop a comprehensive core privileging system for your hospital, see *Core Privileging: A Practical Approach to Development and Implementation*, 2nd edition, published by HCPro, Inc.

Figure 4.1 **Policy and procedure for delineating clinical privileges**

Policy

Requests for clinical privileges will be processed only when the potential applicant meets the board's current minimum threshold criteria. Potential applicants who do not meet these criteria will not have their applications submitted to the medical staff credentials committee and the department chair(s) for evaluation. In the event there is a request for which there are no approved criteria, the board must determine whether it will allow the privilege. If the board allows the privilege, it will use the following procedure to develop criteria. Requests for which the board has approved no specific criteria within 90 days will be processed using the general criteria of adequate education, training, clinical experience, and references demonstrating current clinical competence.

Procedure for developing privilege criteria

Whenever a privileging question arises for which there are no applicable criteria, the credentials committee will follow these steps to coordinate the development of applicable criteria:

1. Develop a research paper concerning the privileging issue to determine how the institution handles the issue at the present time, the possible specialty/subspecialties that may be interested in the issue, the positions held by specialty societies or academies concerning the issue (if any), the type of practitioner(s) who already performs/treats the issue in other similar hospitals, and any other relevant issues.

2. Submit the results of its research to, and seek the opinion of, an ad hoc task force composed of subject matter experts. One of the following mechanisms may be used:

   • A representative of the credentials committee will facilitate a multispecialty group of physicians with a true interest (and knowledge of) the issue
   • The credentials committee will request each individual department/subspecialty to provide it with advice concerning the clinical issue.

3. The ad hoc task force shall have approximately 15 days to advise the credentials committee about

---

Figure 4.1 | **Policy and procedure for delineating clinical privileges (cont.)**

---

the following prerequisites as they relate to each privilege request:

- The type of basic education and, if necessary, continuing education
- The number of years of formal training, and in what field(s) (and, if applicable, continuing training—either didactic or hands-on)

Note: The required number of years of basic residency training may vary by specialty, as might the need for postgraduate continuing medical education/training.

The ad hoc task force that is advising the credentials committee should indicate the required evidence of training if the applicant's postgraduate residency program did not include training in the new procedure (disease). If the task force determines this issue might be relevant, it should indicate the following:

- Whether some years of fellowship should follow completion of an approved residency program
- Whether completion of an approved residency training program should be followed by at least [*insert number*] hours of approved post-graduate training in a university or other educational setting
- Whether prior experience is required and if so, the amount of recent direct or indirect (but applicable) experience (evidence of prior experience may include general hospital experience in the specialty during the past 12 months and/or specific experience in the diagnosis/procedure during the past 12 months).

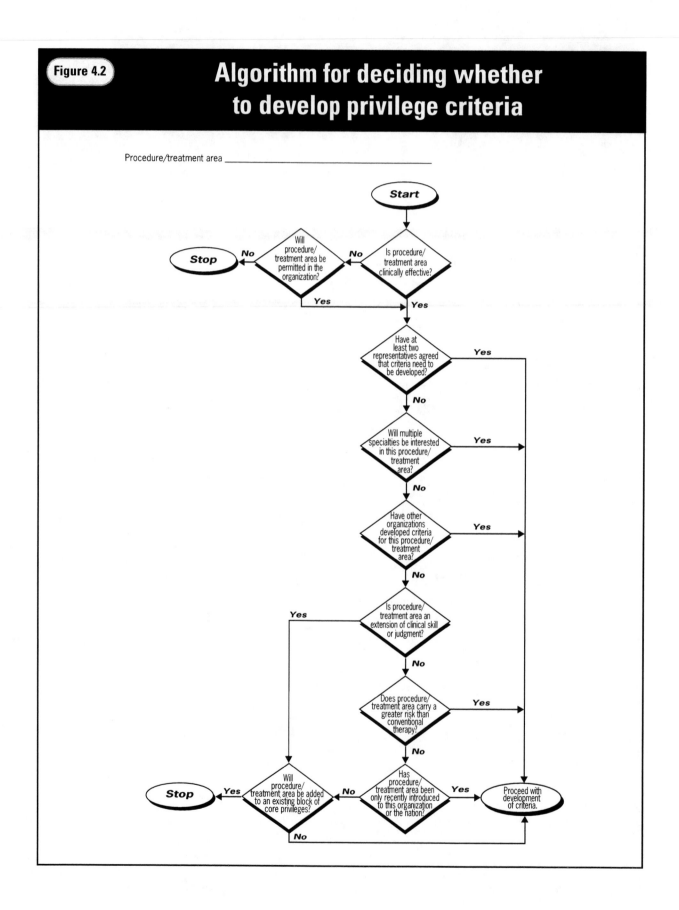

Figure 4.2

Algorithm for deciding whether to develop privilege criteria

Procedure/treatment area _____

Figure 4.3

Worksheet for developing privilege criteria

One form should be finalized for each area in which privileges are requested or granted—either by general category or specific privilege (e.g., core medical privileges, sigmoidoscopies, insertion and management of pulmonary artery catheters).

When a privilege crosses specialty designation and controversy exists, this form should be drafted by each involved specialty and submitted to the medical executive committee for final adjudication.

Instructions

State the amount of education, training, and experience that is (in your opinion) necessary to engage in the specific clinical activity under your consideration. List all possible combinations of qualifications (i.e., if general surgery is drafting criteria for hysterectomy, it should indicate that four years of either general surgery or obstetrical training are required).

Please determine

1. the degree that the successful applicant must have (MD, DO, DDS, DPM)
2. number of years of accredited postgraduate residency or fellowship training is required, and in which programs
3. whether the applicant must be board certified/board admissible
4. how much recent direct or indirect experience in the procedure, illness or disorder, or related field (within the past 12–24 months) the applicant must demonstrate
5. how many and the type of references required to permit evaluation of ability, judgment, and current competence

Note: If a particular category is not required, indicate with "N/A" (not applicable).

Unless otherwise specified

- all required education must have taken place in an institution approved[1] by a national or international organization.
- all training must have taken place in a postgraduate training program accredited[2] by either the AMA, AOA, APMA, AAOMS.
- all experience must have occurred within the past 12 months in an institution with formal performance monitoring improvement programs (organizations accredited by the JCAHO or the AOA are deemed to meet this requirement).
- references must be responsive to the hospital's request and (if provided) returned on a form specified by the hospital.

| Figure 4.3 | Worksheet for developing privilege criteria (cont.) |

Recommended criteria

Privilege(s) in question: _____

Effective dates: _____ to _____

Education

❏ MD   ❏ DO   ❏ DDS   ❏ DPM

Other special education course: _____

_____

Training

_____ years of approved postgraduate training in _____ or

_____.

Fellowship/Board status/Other (if applicable)

Required in _____ or _____.

Experience

Performance of _____ during the past _____ months.

Specifications: _____

_____

References

❏ Not required   ❏ Required

Specifications: _____

_____

[1] For the purposes of this book, an approved institution is one fully accredited throughout the time of the practitioner's attendance by the liaison committee on medical education by the American Osteopathic Association or by the American Dental Association.

[2] An accredited postgraduate training program, fully accredited throughout the time of the practitioner's training.

Figure 4.4

Policy regarding approval of clinical privileges criteria

This hospital will process requests for clinical privileges only when the applicant meets the hospital's minimum threshold criteria. The board hereby delegates the approval function for such criteria as follows:

- Criteria that are applicable to a single-specialty issue for which no controversy exists shall be approved by the credentials committee

- Criteria that are applicable to a multi-specialty issue for which no controversy exists shall be approved by the credentials committee

- Criteria for which there is disagreement among department chairs, but for which no minority report has been submitted shall be approved by the medical executive committee (MEC).

- Criteria for which a minority report has been submitted must be recommended by the MEC and may be approved by the hospital's chief executive officer.

Potential or alleged conflicts of interest will be responded to in the following manner:

- Members of either the credentials committee or MEC who have a potential or alleged conflict of interest will be permitted to participate in committee discussions, but will recuse themselves for the committee's final deliberations and vote.

- If a department chair disagrees with criteria that have been finalized and approved by the credentials committee, he or she may submit a minority report to the MEC. The minority report must include both the department chair's specific objection(s) to the criteria and his or her recommendation for modifying the criteria. When possible, the department chair should support his or her recommendation with references to medical literature, specialty society guidelines, or other definitive evidence suggesting that a different set of criteria relative to education, training, or experience might be more appropriate.

| Figure 4.5 | Policy regarding approval of clinical privileges |

Exercise of privileges

Any practitioner who provides clinical services at this hospital may exercise only those privileges the governing board granted him or her, and emergency privileges as described herein.

Privileges requests

Each applicant must include in his or her application for appointment or reappointment to the medical staff a request for the specific clinical privileges that he or she seeks. An applicant must submit specific requests if he or she wishes to obtain temporary privileges or if he or she seeks modification of privileges in the interim between reappraisals.

Basis for privileges delineation

The hospital will consider a request for clinical privileges only when the request includes evidence of

- education
- training
- experience
- demonstrated current competence (as specified by the hospital)

If the hospital has no threshold criteria for a requested privilege, the hospital will table the request for a reasonable period of time during which the board—after consulting with the credentials committee and MEC—will formulate the necessary criteria. Once the board has established threshold criteria for the requested privilege, the hospital will process the original request.

The hospital will evaluate valid requests for clinical privileges on the basis of

- prior and continuing education
- training
- experience
- utilization practice patterns

Figure 4.5

Policy regarding approval
of clinical privileges (cont.)

- current ability to perform the privileges requested
- demonstrated current competence, ability, and judgment

The hospital might also consider patient care needs, its facility's capability to support the type of privileges being requested, and the availability of qualified coverage in the applicant's absence.

The decision to grant privileges at reappointment or to grant a requested change in privileges must consider

- observed clinical performance
- documented results of the staff's quality improvement program activities
- pertinent information from other sources—especially other institutions and health care settings in which professionals exercise clinical privileges

When processing requests for clinical privileges, the hospital will follow the procedure for granting medical staff membership that is described in the Initial Appointment Policy.

Special conditions

Dental privileges: The hospital will process requests for dental privileges in the same manner as it processes all other privilege requests. Surgical procedures performed by dentists/oral surgeons will be under the overall supervision of the chair of the department of surgery. Every dental patient will receive a basic medical appraisal by a physician member of the medical staff; the result of this appraisal will be recorded in the patient's medical record. Both the physician and the patient's dentist must assess the risks of any proposed procedure and the procedure's potential effect(s) on the patient's health.

The hospital may grant an oral surgeon the privilege of performing history and physicals on his or her patients if he or she submits documentation of completion of an accredited postgraduate residency in oral/maxillofacial surgery and demonstrated current competence.

Figure 4.5

Policy regarding approval
of clinical privileges (cont.)

A physician member of the medical staff will be responsible for the overall medical care of the patient, including care of any medical problems that are present at admission or that arise during hospitalization. The physician must agree to any surgical procedure performed on the patient. "Dental" as used in this policy does not necessarily include oral surgeons.

Allied health professionals: The hospital will process requests from allied health professionals to perform specified patient care services in the manner specified in the policies governing allied health professionals. An allied health professional may, subject to any licensure requirements or other limitations, exercise independent judgment only within the areas of his or her professional competence and participate directly in the medical management of patients under the supervision of a physician who has been accorded privileges to provide such care.

Pediatric privileges: The hospital will process requests for pediatric privileges in the same manner as it processes all other privilege requests. Surgical procedures performed by podiatrists will be under the overall supervision of the chair of the department of surgery. All pediatric patients will receive a basic medical appraisal by a physician member of the medical staff. The results of the appraisal will be recorded in the patient's medical record.

Figure 4.6 — Request for temporary privileges

Please note that this hospital will only grant temporary privileges for the following circumstances as set forth in our General Policy on Clinical Privileges—i.e., to fulfill an important patient-care need (as defined below and in the attached policy) for initial appointment and reappointment, and when an initial applicant with a complete clean application awaits review and approval of the medical executive committee and the governing body.

Applicant name: _____

I hereby request temporary privileges due to the following circumstances (please be as specific as possible):

_____
_____
_____
_____

I understand all conditions associated with this request as specified in the medical staff bylaws and credentialing policies and procedures. I have read these documents and agree to be bound by the terms contained therein.

_____   _____
Applicant's signature   Date

Department Chair's Recommendation:

I recommend that _____, who has applied for [appointment/ reappointment] to the medical staff of this hospital, be granted temporary privileges for a period of _____as requested/modified because of the following important patient care need (check all that apply):

❏ One or more individual patients will experience care that does not adequately meet their clinical needs if the temporary privileges under consideration are not granted (i.e., a patient scheduled for urgent surgery who would not be able to undergo the surgery in a timely manner.)

| Figure 4.6 | Request for temporary privileges (cont.) |

❑The hospital will be placed at risk of not adequately meeting the needs of patients who seek care from the hospital if the temporary privileges under consideration are not granted (i.e., the hospital will not be able to provide adequate emergency room coverage in the provider's specialty).

❑ A group of patients in the community served by the hospital will be placed at risk of not receiving care that meets their clinical needs if the temporary privileges under consideration are not granted (i.e., a physician who has a large practice in the community for which adequate coverage of hospital care for those patients cannot be arranged).

Rationale for the above patient care need determination:

_____

_____

_____

_____

I affirm that I have personally reviewed the appointment/reappointment application of the above-referenced practitioner and have determined that this individual meets the medical staff's criteria for the privileges for which I am recommending temporary privileges. The basis for this determination and how it was verified is as follows:

1. License: _____

2. Area of clinical practice (i.e., emergency medicine): _____

3. Experience: _____

4. Current clinical competence:

_____

_____

Figure 4.6   **Request for temporary privileges (cont.)**

5. Capacity to perform:

_____

_____

Completion of form by:

_____

Department chair, signature

_____

Date

_____

Approved by chief executive officer/president

_____

Date

Note: The second half of this form, which describes how staff determine and verify the required criteria for applicants, may be filled out by the medical staff services professional, if appropriate, with input from the department chair. The medical staff services professional may fill out lines 1–3, and the department chair must fill out lines 4–5. Don't forget to send a copy of this form to the departments that must know who holds temporary privileges, such as the admitting and emergency departments, the operating room, etc.

Figure 4.7   ## Procedure for processing clinical privileges requests

The medical staff coordinator or administrative representative will be responsible for ensuring that each applicant for medical staff appointment or allied health professional (AHP) receives the appropriate privileges request forms.

The privileges request forms should accompany the application and should include the following:

• The hospital's privileges delineation overview

• Instructions for competing the privileges request forms

• Privileges threshold criteria

• The appropriate requested section (e.g., an internist will receive internal medicine forms)

• A special procedures section (if applicable)

All requests for clinical privileges must be submitted, with supporting material, to the medical staff coordinator or administrative representative, who will do the following:

1. Verify the supporting material

2. Compile current privileges (if any) and administrative review (if any) with the application *(Note: This section routinely applies only to current medical staff appointees who are requesting additional clinical privilege.)*

3. Make two copies of the completed privileges request package: one for the file, and another for the applicable department chair

4. Submit the application package, with supporting material, to the applicable department chair

---

Figure 4.7

Procedure for processing clinical privileges requests (cont.)

The department chair will do the following:

1. Review the request and all supporting material against threshold criteria for granting clinical privileges and, where necessary, conduct a personal clinical interview with the requestor

2. Formulate a written report and forward it to the credentials committee

If the credentials committee's recommendation is positive, the medical staff coordinator or administrative representative will send a letter to the applicant, signed by the applicable department chair, regarding any special conditions/observation requirements.

Once the medical executive committee/governing board approves the credentials committee's recommendation, the chief executive officer will notify the applicant of his or her new privileges.

Figure 4.8

Department chair's report and recommendation on privileges request(s)

[*Date*]

Applicant: [*Practitioner name*]

Specialty: [*Name—i.e., Orthopedic Surgery*]

Privileges requested in:

    A. Department of [*Name department/section (i.e., Department of Medicine, Section of Cardiology)*]
    B. Department of [*Name department/section*]
    C. Department of [*Name department/section*]

I have reviewed the above-referenced practitioner's file including the supporting documentation for the privileges requested.

    A. Based upon my review, I find that the applicant is qualified for the privileges listed on the attached sheet. My specific findings are as follows:

	Adequate	Inadequate**
Education	❏	❏
Training	❏	❏
Experience	❏	❏
Evidence of current clinical competence	❏	❏
Health status*	❏	❏
Additionally, the criteria for privileges review have been met.	❏	❏

    B. I am unable to formulate a report for the following reasons:

    _____

    _____

    C. **My finding is unfavorable due to inadequate education, training, experience, or references (see file), specifically:

    _____

    _____

_____   _____

Department chair signature   **Date**

All organizations must comply with the Americans with Disabilities Act.

Figure 4.9 Request for modification of clinical privileges

All requests for increased privileges must be accompanied by information demonstrating current clinical competence in the privileges requested. Information should be supplied (original form) demonstrating the education, training, and experience you believe qualifies you for the privileges. One letter from a recognized expert in the clinical discipline involved should be submitted as well.

I hereby request additional clinical privileges as follows (or see attached).

A. _____

B. _____

C. _____

D. _____

E. _____

I have attached full details demonstrating my competence in these areas.

_____

Appointee's signature

_____

Date

Chapter 5

Quality Data

for

Reappointment

Quality Data for Reappointment

The language of the Joint Commission on Accreditation of Healthcare Organizations' (JCAHO) reappointment standards seems so benign: It requires all medical staffs and boards to appoint physicians to the medical staff for a period of no more than two years. It also requires that the criteria for privileges include evidence of current competence. These two deceptively simple requirements lead to one huge challenge for medical staffs and the quality and medical staff services professionals who support them: How do we determine current competence at the time of reappointment?

To answer this challenge, we must solve the "competency equation". You can write the competency equation in the following manner:

$$\text{Current competence} = \frac{\text{Evidence that you've done ``X'' recently}}{\text{When you did ``X,'' did you do it well?}}$$

"X" in this equation refers to whatever the physician does for which we are attempting to assess current competence. The X may be a specific procedure, management of a particular clinical condition, or a collection of conditions and procedures.

The competency equation, along with relevant regulatory requirements, makes it necessary to generate a report at the time of reappointment that fills in the two variables in this equation. In other words, the two variables are the data reviewed by department chairs, the credentials committee and the medical executive committee (MEC) at the time of reappointment must include measures of the practitioner's clinical activity since the last reappointment time as well as measures of how well the practitioner has carried out those clinical activities. Together, these constitute a physician performance profile. It is this physician performance profile that physician leaders must count on in deciding what recommendation to make regarding a reapplicant's request for membership and privileges.

Evidence that you've done 'X' recently?

To answer this question, your information management systems must be able to produce a report of clinical activity specific to each physician at the time of reappointment. If your systems cannot produce such a report, you will have to resort to manually gathering this information, which can be very time consuming. You also know what your next request of your IT department will be.

Assuming your systems can produce a physician-specific clinical activity report, you must decide how you want this information organized. This decision will depend upon the method your medical staff has selected for delineating privileges. The two most common methods for delineating privileges today are procedure and condition specific lists (frequently called "laundry lists") and core privileges.[1]

If your medical staff uses laundry lists, then the best way to organize and display your data is according to the specific procedures and conditions in each specialty's privilege form. Organizing and displaying data in this manner provides the best support to department chairs, the credentials committee and the MEC as they attempt to answer the first question—has the physician done X lately. X in this case refers to each privilege on the laundry list.

If your medical staff delineates privileges by using core privileges and special procedure requests, then organizing physician profile data relative to privileges is more straightforward. When core privileges are well-designed, your medical staff will have previously established criteria for eligibility to request the core as well as eligibility to request each special privilege. The core for each specialty should be described clearly enough so the physician's activity that falls within the core is easy to identify from your information systems that track physician clinical activity. This allows you to organize the physician performance report by care (including admissions, procedures and consults) that falls within the core and care that involves each of the specially requested privileges outside of the core. Then volume for each specially requested privilege can be tracked separately.

Volume makes a difference

Physicians fall into three volume categories at the time of reappointment:
- Category 1: Active at your hospital
- Category 2: Little activity at your hospital, but active at another hospital
- Category 3: Little activity at any hospital, including yours

For category 1 physicians, it is relatively easy to answer the question, "Have you done 'it' recently?" Generate a report from your own information systems that tracks physician-specific

---

[1] *If you are not familiar with core privileges, you may find more details about it in* Core Privileges: A Practical Approach to Development and Implementation, Second Edition. *Bob Gillesby, Hugh P. Greeley, Beverly Pybus, CMSC, Richard Sheff. 2003. HCPro Inc. Marblehead, MA.*

volume in the manner most appropriate to how privileges are delineated. (Of course this report will only be as good as your current information systems allow, but that is a different kind of challenge.)

Category 2 physicians are somewhat more challenging, because you have little information from your own systems that can answer the "Have you done 'it' recently?" question. So category 2 physicians must depend upon information gathered by other hospitals. Category 3 physicians are even more challenging.

Does recent volume matter?

Most physicians are very uncomfortable addressing the issue of whether recent volume matters in assessing and determining current competence. Many physicians believe that if they were once competent at a particular procedure or managing a clinical condition, they always will be. This is simply not true. Some aspects of practicing medicine are like riding a bicycle, meaning physician performance doesn't decay over time if they haven't done it. Other aspects of practicing medicine do decay over time. These may result in a decline in technique, or not having the right reflexes in a rapidly evolving emergency.

Because medical skills can deteriorate over time, only the medical staff can determine which privileges will be considered like riding a bicycle and which require evidence of recent volume.

Does volume correlate with competence?

Some physicians claim that competence does not correlate with volume. The American Academy of Family Practice (AAFP) has publicly taken the position that the competence of each physician should be established on a case-by-case basis, without threshold volume criteria for eligibility. The correlation of volume with clinical outcomes is well established in research for relatively few procedures. And sometimes the correlation of clinical outcomes is with the entire team's volume, not just the individual physician's volume. However, in each circumstance in which it has been adequately studied, clinical outcomes have been shown to correlate with at least a minimum-volume threshold. But whether you embrace the position of the AAFP or a position that minimum threshold volumes should be established and enforced, your medical staff must ultimately develop an answer to the question, "Have you done 'X' recently?"

When you did 'X,' did you do it well?

Once your systems have gathered data that answers the question of whether a physician has done "X", medical staff leaders require data that answers the question, "Have you done 'it' well?" JCAHO requires that decisions regarding privileges include criteria of license, training, experience, current competence and the capacity to perform the requested privileges. As a result, at the time of initial appointment and each reappointment, department chairs should be asking whether the applicant meets all of these criteria for each requested privilege. Answering this question for every requested privilege for each physician can be a very daunting task given the wide range of clinical activities in which most of them engage. In fact, it is never done. Instead, department chairs assume that "no news is good news". In other words, if the physician has not had blatantly poor results in peer review or been responsible for major sentinel events since the last appointment time, the physician is deemed to be competent in the privileges granted the last time. This means that at reappointment, the average physician assumes he or she will be granted the same privileges as before unless the hospital can prove the physician is incompetent.

This approach stands credentialing and privileging on its head. Instead, the burden should be placed on physicians to demonstrate that they meet the hospital's criteria for license, training, experience, current competence and capacity to perform all the privileges requested. But the hospital is responsible for tracking data on care provided within the hospital. So the burden placed on the applicant should apply to care provided outside of the hospital. For care provided within the hospital, physician leaders should decide what data should be collected to solve the competency equation in the affirmative, not just the absence of bad news.

So if your medical staff is still using laundry lists, determining current competence would require a department chair to review data on the physician's performance of each privilege requested. Since this is obviously unrealistic, the next best approach would be for each department to identify a hierarchy of privileges within their specialty from most complex to least complex. If physicians demonstrate good clinical outcomes in the most complex privileges, they would be deemed competent to carry out the less complex privileges. An example of such a hierarchy for intra-abdominal procedures in general surgery is found in Figure 5.1, located at the end of this chapter. From this example, you can see that a physician who demonstrates competence in complex procedures, such as surgical treatment of the acute abdomen, colectomy, or laparoscopic cholecystectomy with common bile duct exploration and repair, would be deemed competent to perform simpler procedures such as lysis of adhesions, simple laparoscopic cholecystectomy, and incisional hernia repair.

You can see how complex a challenge it is to develop a hierarchy such as this for each specialty. This is another reason core privileging makes more sense than laundry lists. For core privileging, the first "X" in the competency equation refers to the core itself. To establish competency within the core, the data need only show that the physician has successfully provided care across a reasonably representative sample of clinical activities included in the core. This is logistically far easier, and more statistically valid, than tracking outcomes by each privilege requested by each physician. For the few specially requested procedures, outcome data would be required which is procedure or diagnosis specific. A sample of a physician performance report organized by surgical core privileges is found in Figure 5.2.

Finally, it is important to recognize because of how peer review is practiced at most hospitals, the data that we currently obtain from it is very limited. Peer review generally involves reviewing individual charts of cases that "fall out" based on screening criteria that are designed to identify when something bad happens. However, most medical staffs review large numbers of charts, yet in only a few cases do they ever conclude that the physician didn't meet the standard of care. So physician performance profiles that depend primarily on the results of peer review of individual charts will have remarkably little data at the time or reappointment for most physicians.

The Greeley Measurement Method

The Greeley Measurement Method has been developed to address this lack of data. In this method, medical staff indicators are divided in to three types, called Types 1, 2 and 3.

Type 1 indicators
Type 1 indicators evaluate rules violations. Samples of such rules include the following:

- We don't transfuse medically stable patients with a hemoglobin greater than 8
- A history and physical must be on the patient's chart prior to surgery
- Peak and trough gentamycin levels should be drawn before and after the fifth dose
- All entries in the medical record must be legible

If a physician violates one of these rules, he or she would receive immediate feedback and a reminder about the rule in order to enable him or her to self-correct. The rule violation would also be entered into a database. At reappointment time, this data can be turned into a report. Physicians would have to become comfortable in using this data, so any single violation is not held against a physician. At reappointment time, the department chair, credentials committee and MEC would only be interested in physicians who repeatedly violate rules and do not demonstrate improvement after receiving feedback on their violation of such rules.

Type 2 indicators
Type 2 indicators are significant events. These are major patient injuries or adverse outcomes that require evaluation of the chart to determine the cause and severity. The goal of evaluating such cases is to determine whether the physician demonstrated the adequate fund of knowledge, skill, and judgment to carry out the privileges granted. At reappointment time there should be relatively few examples of such cases. Again, a single case with adverse findings in peer review does not

warrant limiting a physician's privileges unless the case clearly demonstrates significant physician deficits. Instead, a pattern of providing care that does not meet the accepted standard of care would be the type of finding that would lead to concerns about a physician's competence.

Type 3 indicators

Type 3 indicators are rates. These involve a numerator and denominator. Examples of rates relevant to assessing current competence might include the following:

- Unintended organ injury rates during surgery or other procedures
- Compliance rate with the approved anticoagulation protoco
- Frequency of Apgar scores less than 7 at five minutes
- Rate of compliance with core measures, such as aspirin and beta-blockers in myocardial infarction and angiotensin converting enzyme inhibitors in chronic heart failure

This rate-based data should be continuously tracked and fed back to physicians so they have a chance to self-correct. It should also allow for appreciation of physicians who perform well on these indicators. At the time of reappointment, the physician and his or her department chair will already know this data. It is some of the most helpful data in determining current competence at the time of reappointment. An example of a core privileges based physician performance profile using The Greeley Measurement Method is found in Figure 5.3.

Don't use reappointment to play 'gotcha'

A final word of caution is warranted here. Physician performance data at the time of reappointment should not be a surprise. Unfortunately, reappointment is frequently the first time data on a particular physician's performance is pulled together into a coherent picture of that physician's performance. At reappointment time, we are considering modifying a physician's membership or privileges based on past performance. This makes it a very high-stakes time—and a very defensive time—for physicians. It also doesn't give the physician a chance to self-correct prior to his or her membership or privileges being in jeopardy.

The best approach is to provide periodic performance reports to physicians, at least annually and preferably more often. The goal is that physicians use this information to identify and implement opportunities to improve. Department chairs and chiefs of staff might also use these reports to express appreciation to physicians who are performing well and providing excellent care. Periodic honest feedback, both positive and negative, is the best way to treat physicians fairly and stay away from playing "gotcha."

Figure 5.1	Physician performance feedback report: Department of surgery

Open intra-abdominal procedures	Description	Number of cases	Physician-specific performance data
Highly complex	This category includes Whipple procedures, repair of a ruptured viscus, management of penetrating trauma, and other procedures that require a comparable level of knowledge and skill.		
Moderately complex	This category includes bowel resection with anastamosis or colostomy, gastric resection with anastamosis, open cholecystectomy with biliary tree exploration, and other procedures that require a comparable level of knowledge and skill.		
Minimally complex	This category includes open cholecystectomy, open appendectomy, and lysis of adhesions.		
Intra-abdominal laparscopic procedures			
Complex	This category includes complex intra-abdominal laparoscopic procedures such as Nissen fundoplication, complex cholecystectomy with biliary tree exploration, and other procedures that require a comparable level of knowledge and skill.		
Minimally complex	This category includes minimally complex intra-abdominal laparascopic procedures such as closed cholecystectomy, closed appendectomy, and other procedures that require a comparable level of knowledge and skill.		

Figure 5.2	Physician performance feedback report using surgical core privileges

Privileges	Number of cases	Physician-specific performance data
Clinical activities within the core		
Special procedures		
Complex laparascopic procedures		
Bariatric surgery		
Ventilator management beyond 48 hours post-op		
Tracheostomy		
Gastroscopy		
Sentinel node biopsy for cancer		
Use of laser		
Administration of conscious sedation		

Figure 5.3

The Greeley Measurement Method

Privileges	Number of cases	Type 1 results compared to peers	Type 2 results compared to peers	Type 3 results compared to peers
Clinical activities within the core				
Special procedures				
Complex laparascopic procedures				
Bariatric surgery				
Ventilator management beyond 48 hours post-op				
Tracheostomy				
Gastroscopy				
Sentinel node biopsy for cancer				
Use of laser				
Administration of conscious sedation				

Chapter 6

Professional

Review

Action

Professional Review Action

When reviewing physicians' performance feedback reports during the reappointment process, the hospital may determine that he or she has failed to maintain the competence to perform all requested clinical privileges.

When the credentials committee's recommendation is unfavorable to the applicant—either with respect to reappointment or to some or all of the requested clinical privileges—that recommendation is forwarded to the medical executive committee (MEC).

If the credentials committee recommends that the hospital grant the applicant medical staff membership, but deny some of the requested privileges, the applicant has a right to request a hearing, but he or she should also have the option to withdraw his or her request for those privileges.

Under the reporting requirements of the Health Care Quality Improvement Act (HCQIA) of 1986, the withdrawal of the request does not have to be reported to the state medical board; however, if the hospital ultimately denies certain requested privileges, the hospital is obligated to report that denial to the National Practitioner Data Bank (NPDB) via the medical licensing board.

Procedural due process

Remember, although the hospital has the authority and obligation to evaluate medical staff members and prospective members against specific defined criteria and take corrective action when necessary, it must allow a practitioner to challenge an adverse credentialing decision.

Procedural due-process safeguards provide practitioners with mechanisms that ensure fairness and consideration of all relevant competency information. These safeguards allow a practitioner adversely affected by a credentials decision the opportunity to challenge that decision and to present his or her own position. This process must be defined in a fair hearing plan or as provisions in the medical staff bylaws.

Generally, the hospital will retain a lawyer who will represent both the hospital and the medical staff. There may be some instances in which the medical staff organization hires its own lawyer.

Before releasing any information, whether it pertains to an internal investigation or an external request for information or subpoena, it is always advisable to contact the hospital's legal counsel.

Corrective action

The reappointment process requires hospitals to assess the practitioner's clinical performance. During this review, the hospital may decide that corrective action is necessary. Corrective action is the means by which medical staff organizations enforce qualifications and standards and promote professionalism by improving performance.

The following is quoted from attorney Elizabeth Snelson's chapter on corrective action in the book, *Credentialing and Medical Staff Law*, published by the National Association Medical Staff Services:

"Professional competence and conduct" is the term used in the [HCQIA] to describe grounds for professional review actions that give rise to hearing rights and reporting responsibility. The term is defined very generally in the HCQIA: The term "professional review action" means an action or recommendation of a professional review body which is taken or made in the conduct of professional review activity, which is based on the competence or professional conduct of an individual physician (which conduct affects or could affect adversely the health or welfare of a patient or patients), and which affects (or may affect) adversely the clinical privileges, or membership in a professional society, of the physician."

A hospital may also take corrective action to enforce other reappointment requirements, including failure to fully disclose information requested by the medical staff reapplication.

Note: Occasionally a hospital must take corrective action that affects a practitioner's medical staff membership status or clinical privileges in the interim between formal reappointments or before the conclusion of the provisional period. The organization's medical staff bylaws and credentialing procedures manual should detail this process.

The following are the three major levels of action that can be taken:

1. **Corrective action,** where the matter is investigated before any formal action occurs
2. **Summary suspension,** where the potential for harm to patients or others requires the hospital to take immediate action and then the circumstances investigated for withdrawal, continuation, etc.
3. **Automatic action,** where a sanction by an external authority (e.g., licensing board, state or federal drug enforcement agency, federal agency for Medicare/Medicaid sanctions) must automatically result in some type of sanction involving the practitioner's hospital status or practice, or where failure to complete or prepare medical records in timely fashion, after

warning, results in some type of suspension, or failure to maintain the required minimum amount of professional liability insurance, or the coverage is cancelled or not renewed.

The medical staff bylaws or credentialing procedure manual must define the criteria for initiating each type of action and the medical staff/board authorities permitted to initiate the same, as well as the procedures for reaching a final decision on the matter.

The medical staff office personnel's role will vary from hospital to hospital with regard to the corrective action process. As soon as the problem with a practitioner is identified, through the reappointment process of otherwise, the hospital's legal counsel should be contacted and informed of the situation. Legal counsel provides guidance to the medical staff office throughout the process and monitors that the procedural requirements and time frames are met. The medical staff services professional should be familiar with the time requirements in case she or he is called on to track events/to collect various reports and letters.

Fair hearings and appeals

Fair hearings are an unavoidable reality in today's health care environment. According to a 2002 benchmarking survey conducted by **Medical Staff Briefing,** published by HCPro. Inc., in Marble-head, MA, 66% of respondents reported that their medical executive committee recommended disciplinary action against a medical staff member during the last 36 months, and 53% held a fair hearing during the same time period.

Although the Joint Commission on Accreditation of Healthcare Organizations has long required health care organizations to implement a fair hearing and appeals process to address adverse actions taken against medical staff members, the factors that contribute to the complexity of the fair hearing process continue to increase as the health care field becomes more litigious and adversarial.

Assembling an effective fair hearing panel is the key to implementing sound policies to address these factors—i.e., the reasons for conducting a fair hearing, and ways to reduce the need for a fair hearing. It's important that you ensure panel members are educated about their roles and responsibilities, and are aware of potential legal risks.

Because of the time and cost of the fair hearing process, the fair hearing must be equipped to effectively carry out the process and avoid legal pitfalls. During the recent benchmarking survey, 63% of respondents reported that their fair hearings last between one and three days.

However, fair hearings don't always conclude so quickly. In fact 31% of survey respondents reported that their organization had a board appeal in the last 36 months, and 14% of physicians involved in such appeals filed suit against the hospital or the medical staff as a result of a fair hearing finding—further extending the process.

The cost, according to the survey, ranges from under $15,000 (26%) to more than $151,000 (18%) per hearing. And 88% of hospitals participating in the survey do not compensate physicians on the fair hearing panel—further complicating the challenge of finding physicians who will accept appointment to the panel, voluntarily commit the time needed to fulfill their duties, and open

Fair hearing benchmarking survey results

Survey respondents provided the following information regarding fair hearings that took place at their facility in during a 36 month period.

✓ **MEC recommended disciplinary action against a physician**
- *66%*

✓ **Had a fair hearing**
- *53%*

✓ **Number of fair hearing per respondent**
- *28 had one*
- *15 had two*
- *One had 20*

✓ **Number of days fair hearing lasted**
- *One day (35%)*
- *Two to three days (28%)*
- *Four to 10 days (10%)*

Percentage of time the fair hearing panel agreed with the MEC's decision
- *80%*

✓ **Respondents who had a board appeal**
- *31%*

✓ **Hospital sued by medical staff or physician**
- *14%*

✓ **Costs per fair hearing and appeal**
- *$15,000 (26%)*
- *$15,000–$30,000 (18%)*
- *$31,000–$50,000 (16%)*
- *$50,000–$150,000 (18%)*
- *More than $151,000 (18%)*

✓ **Size of medical staff**
- *Less than 100 active members (21%)*
- *101–200 active members (17%)*
- *201–500 active members (42%)*
- *More than 500 active members (20%)*

✓ **Respondents do not compensate panel members**
- *88%*

themselves up to the legal risks associated with hearings. See below for other survey results. Physicians are not only reluctant to sit in judgment of their peers, but many are also concerned about the time involved, the litigation that may ensue, and the politics that surround fair hearing committees. To overcome this reluctance, it's important that you educate your medical staff about the fair hearing process and make certain the members of your fair hearing panel fully understand their roles and responsibilities.

This education should address the following concerns:

Indemnity

Distribute information to your medical staff about the HCQIA and the protections it offers to fair hearing participants. The HCQIA provides immunity to members of the professional body as well as its staff, the hospital in charge of the body, and the people who participate in or assist the professional review body.

However, because a hospital could be sued for defamation or libel if a hearing is not conducted appropriately, and because the HCQIA protects participants from damages but not lawsuits, physicians asked to serve on a fair hearing committee should immediately determine whether the organization will indemnify them if a physician sues the panel for alleged wrongdoing. If a hospital is not willing to indemnify panel members, physicians should think long and hard about serving on the committee. Even though the risk of becoming involved in a suit is fairly low, it nevertheless is still a considerable threat.

The fair hearings plan

Provide the fair hearing panel members with a copy of your organization's medical staff bylaws and fair hearing plan. These documents should identify the responsibilities of the panel members, hospital, and physician under review. The fair hearing plan should also detail the roles of attorneys involved in the process. Panel members should pay particular attention to the investigation and corrective action sections of the fair hearing plan.

In addition to providing the documents mentioned above, hospitals should give physicians on the fair hearing panel an opportunity to meet with the hospital's legal counsel to discuss the process and learn about the panel chair or hearing officer's role.

Role during a fair hearing

Panel members are required to listen, ask questions when necessary for clarification, and work with other panel members to reach a rational and fair conclusion. Generally, panel members are expected to hear the evidence against the physician in support of the MEC recommendation and hear the rebuttal from the physician under review. The burden of demonstrating that the MEC's recommendation is capricious, malicious, or without basis falls on the physician who requests the hearing.

The fair hearing panel members should be warned not to react impulsively to the following claims commonly made by physicians under review:

- The MEC has not suspended other medical staff members who follow the same standard of care or take the same actions as the physician under review. While this may be true, this claim has nothing to do with the validity of the case. Such claims are analogous to the person stopped by a police officer for speeding who claims other drivers were also speeding.

- The MEC's action is a violation of antitrust laws or otherwise illegal. Such allegations often cause the fair hearing panel to question their or the MEC's decision. Stick to the clinical issues and let the attorneys battle about the legality of the action outside of the fair hearing meeting. These meetings are meant to be a discussion among physicians, not a long, complicated discussion of the law.

- The MEC's action was based on the physician's race or gender. Advise the fair hearing panel members that they should focus on the involved clinical issues. Fair hearing panel members should refrain from discussing the consequences of its decision during the fair hearing meeting—for example, reporting the action to the NPDB, the effect of the decision on the practitioner's practice, etc.

Validation of summary suspension decisions

Fair hearing panel members have the difficult job of determining when MEC action is warranted.

Experts advise that panel members should keep in mind the general rule that summary suspension is warranted any time a medical staff officer, or other person empowered to issue a summary suspension, believes that a medical staff member presents a threat to patients, hospital employees, visitors to the facility, or other medical staff members.

Corrective action should not be reserved for patient care decisions that lead to negative outcomes. The purpose of the MEC and fair hearing panel is to prevent care that might subject patients to harm.

In addition, summary suspension may be necessary to carry out an investigation to determine whether the physician can provide safe and effective patient care.

For example, a chief of surgery may be forced to suspend a surgeon accused of intoxication. If immediate investigation reveals that the surgeon is not intoxicated, the precautionary suspension should be lifted. However, if immediate investigation reveals that the surgeon is intoxicated, the suspension should be maintained pending the MEC's final resolution.

Note: In some cases, a single incident may be enough to warrant corrective action. In such extreme cases—such as a physician abandoning a critically ill patient to attend to a personal matter—the hospital's decision to suspend that physician is often justified.

Figure 6.1 — **Routine investigation procedure**

Requests and notices

All requests for investigation must be in writing, submitted to or created by the medical executive committee (MEC), and supported by references to specific activities or conduct that constitute grounds for the request. The chief of staff must promptly notify the chief executive officer of the investigation request.

Investigation

After deliberation, the MEC may either act on a request immediately or require that an investigation takes place. The MEC may conduct an investigation itself, or assign this task to a medical staff officer, department, ad hoc committee, or other organizational component.

The investigative process does not follow the same steps as the hospital's fair hearing plan. However, it may involve consultations with the practitioner, the individual or group making the request, and other individuals who may have knowledge of relevant events.

If the investigation is conducted by a group or individual other than the MEC, that group or individual must forward a written report of the investigation to the MEC as soon as possible. The MEC may terminate the investigation process at any time, at its discretion or at the request of the governing board, and may proceed with action as provided below.

MEC action

The MEC acts upon a request for investigation within 60 days of the receipt of the request, unless deferred. Its action may include recommending

- rejection of the request for investigation

- a warning, formal letter, or reprimand

- a probationary period with retrospective review of cases, without special requirements for concurrent consultation or direct supervision

- suspension of appointment prerogatives that do not affect clinical privileges

---

Figure 6.1

Routine investigation procedure (cont.)

- individual requirements for consultation or supervision

- reduction, suspension, or revocation of clinical privileges

- suspension or limitation of prerogatives directly related to the practitioner's provision of patient care

- suspension or revocation of staff appointment

- any other action believed to be in the best interest of patient care and safety

Deferral

The MEC may defer action if additional time is needed to complete the investigation. A subsequent recommendation for one or more of the actions provided above must be made within nine days of the deferral.

Procedural rights

An MEC recommendation for individual concurring consultation, decreased privileges, diminished or suspended patient care prerogatives, or suspended or revoked appointment is deemed adverse and entitles the practitioner to the procedural rights contained in the fair hearing plan.

An MEC recommendation for rejection, diminished prerogatives not affecting clinical privileges, a warning or reprimand, or probation with retrospective monitoring are not deemed adverse and should be submitted to the governing board with all supporting documentation.

Figure 6.2 — Investigation and corrective action policy

Behavior leading to initiation of an investigation

Routine investigation: An investigation may be initiated whenever a practitioner with clinical privileges exhibits behavior—either within or outside the hospital—that is likely to be detrimental to the quality of patient care or safety, the hospital's operations, or the community's confidence in the hospital.

A routine investigation may be initiated by any medical staff officer, the chair of the department in which the practitioner holds appointment or exercises clinical privileges, the chief executive officer (CEO), the medical executive committee, or the governing board.

Interviews prior to an investigation and corrective action

An individual or committee considering initiating an investigation or corrective action may arrange for an interview with the involved practitioner. During the interview, circumstances prompting the consideration of investigation or corrective action are discussed, and the practitioner is asked to present relevant information on his or her own behalf. A written record reenacting the substance of the interview is maintained, and copies are sent to the practitioner, chief of staff, and CEO.

If the practitioner fails or declines to participate in the interview, the appropriate investigation or corrective action is initiated. According to the procedural rules provided in the fair hearing plan, an interview is not a practitioner's procedural right and need not be conducted.

Automatic suspension

Automatic suspension shall be initiated in the following circumstances:

1. Whenever a practitioner's state license or DEA number is revoked, suspended, restricted, or placed under probation
2. Whenever a practitioner fails to satisfy an interview requirement
3. Whenever a practitioner fails to maintain malpractice insurance
4. Whenever a practitioner's medical records are not completed in a timely manner

State license

Revocation: Whenever a practitioner's license to practice in this state is revoked, his or her medical staff appointment and clinical privileges are immediately and automatically revoked.

Figure 6.2 — Investigation and corrective action policy (cont.)

Restriction: Whenever a practitioner's license is partially limited or restricted, his or her clinical privileges are similarly limited or restricted.

Suspension: Whenever a practitioner's license is suspended, his or her staff appointment and clinical privileges are automatically suspended, effective upon and for at least the term of the suspension.

Probation: Whenever a practitioner is placed on probation by a licensing agency, his or her voting and office-holding prerogatives are automatically suspended, effective upon and for at least the term of the probation.

Drug enforcement

Whenever a practitioner's right to prescribe controlled substances is revoked, restricted, suspended, or placed on probation by a licensing authority (i.e., DEA), his or her privileges to prescribe such substances in the hospital will also be revoked, restricted, suspended, or placed on probation automatically and to the same degree. This will be effective upon and for at least the term of the imposed restriction.

Medical records preparation and completion

The medical staff rules and regulations outline the rules for medical records preparation and completion. The rules call for an automatic suspension of all of a practitioner's clinical privileges if his or her operative reports are not dictated within 24 hours or if a medical record is not completed within a 14-day period from when the practitioner was notified and the record was made available.

Timely completion: A practitioner's failure to prepare/complete medical records in a timely fashion may result in the limitation or automatic suspension of some or all of his or her prerogatives and clinical privileges. This will not occur without sufficient time and written warning and so will not constitute a hardship.

Voluntary resignation: Six suspensions within any 12-month period for failure to complete or prepare records will be deemed a voluntary resignation from the staff. Practitioners who so resign may immediately submit a formal application for reappointment.

Professional liability insurance

A practitioner who fails to maintain a minimum amount of professional liability insurance will have his or her medical staff appointment and clinical privileges immediately suspended.

Figure 6.2 Investigation and corrective action policy (cont.)

Medical executive committee (MEC) recommendation

After a practitioner's license is suspended, restricted, or placed on probation, or after his or her controlled substances registration is revoked, restricted, suspended, or placed on probation, the MEC convenes as soon as possible to review and consider the facts under which action was taken. The MEC may then recommend further corrective action as is appropriate to the facts disclosed in the investigation, including limitation of prerogatives.

Further action

The procedures for further action on an investigation are contained in the fair hearing plan.

Summary suspension

The CEO or any member of the MEC or the governing board may initiate summary suspension. They have the authority to summarily suspend a practitioner's medical staff status or any portion of clinical privileges. The CEO is to give prompt special notice of the summary suspension, which is effective immediately, to the practitioner.

Summary suspension shall be initiated whenever a practitioner's conduct requires that immediate action be taken to prevent immediate danger to life, or injury to him or herself, patients, employees, or other persons present in the hospital.

The appropriate department chair must assign a suspended practitioner's hospitalized patient to another practitioner. When feasible, the chair should consider the patient's wishes in choosing a substitute practitioner.

MEC action

As soon as possible (generally within 72 hours after a summary suspension has been imposed), the MEC will convene to review and consider the suspension. The MEC may recommend modification, continuation, or termination of the suspension terms.

Procedural rights

Unless the MEC recommends the suspension be immediately terminated or modified to one of the lesser sanctions outlined herein, the practitioner is entitled to the procedural rights contained in the fair hearing plan.

Figure 6.2 **Investigation and corrective action policy (cont.)**

Other action

An MEC recommendation to terminate or modify the suspension to a lesser sanction, thereby not triggering procedural rights, is transmitted immediately, with all supporting documentation, to the governing board. In this instance, the MEC's recommendation will revoke the summary suspension completely, or reinstate the practitioner with whatever corrective action the MEC assessed before the governing board's final decision.

Reapplication subsequent to corrective correction

An applicant who has been denied appointment, clinical privileges, or reappointment, or who has been removed from the medical staff during the appointment year, may not reapply to this hospital for a period of one year (12 months), unless specified otherwise in the terms of the specific corrective action.

Chapter 7

Non-Active and Low-Volume Physicians:

A recurring problem

Non-Active and Low-Volume Physicians: A recurring problem

Credentialing professionals often dread reappointment time for physicians who work very little or not at all in the hospital. It's nearly impossible to collect quality and outcomes data on them: Quality improvement, risk management, and other departments compile very little information, if any, on these practitioners. But because the Joint Commission on Accreditation of Healthcare Organizations (JCAHO) requires hospitals to base their reappointment and privileging recommendations on evidence of physicians' current clinical competence (**MS.5.15** in the Medical Staff chapter of the *Comprehensive Accreditation Manual for Hospitals*), they must develop policies and procedures for obtaining necessary data for so-called "low-volume providers." The suggestions below may help to solve this dilemma.

Non-active physicians

Many hospitals struggle with non-active physicians who continually reapply to the medical staff. In most of these situations, the physicians have no intention of helping the medical staff with its clinical work or medical staff membership duties such as emergency department coverage, committee service, charity cases, education, etc. They simply want to add the reappointment to their curriculum vitae or to facilitate working with a health maintenance organization. Also, some physicians fear that if they give up their appointment, they will not be able to regain it in the future.

But make no mistake, these practitioners aren't internists or family physicians who practice exclusively in ambulatory care settings and refer patients to the hospital. They are physicians who have no intention of admitting, consulting, referring, or participating in medical staff matters in any way.

How can hospitals discover a non-active practitioner's intentions? They could include a short questionnaire or "intended practice plan" as part of the reappointment package. Today, more and more medical staffs ask initial applicants to complete an intended practice plan—a form on which they document their intended commitment to the hospital, medical staff, emergency department, and, in some instances, the surrounding community. The hospital will cease to process the applications of physicians who indicate their unwillingness to provide emergency care, participate in medical staff activities, use the hospital for inpatient care, refer their outpatients to the institution, or otherwise assist the hospital in living up to its mission. Such a move should not involve a denial of membership/privileges, shame, blame, or a fair-hearing process. By not processing the application in the first place, hospitals avoid these pitfalls.

By the same token, when practitioners up for reappointment clearly indicate no interest in the hospital or its mission, one solution might be to cease the reapplication process. Another solution might be to grant very short conditional or limited reappointments that could be extended once the practitioner "makes good" on his or her promise to help the medical staff and hospital with its clinical work.

Other hospitals take a different approach to this problem. Specifically, they require very high dues for physicians who do not assist the medical staff. Still others institute a reapplication fee for non-active physicians, reappoint without granting privileges, or withhold reapplications from physicians with no involvement at the facility for the past four years.

Low-volume physicians

When determining how to handle low-volume providers, medical staff leaders and medical staff professionals alike should steer clear of common privileging myths. These myths prevent hospitals from developing policies and procedures that place the burden on the physician to provide competency data. For example, hospitals shouldn't be blinded by past practices. In other words, just because a physician used to perform a certain procedure all the time "way back when" does not mean he or she is still competent to perform that procedure today. If a physician requests privileges for a procedure that he or she has not performed in the hospital often (or at all), the hospital should obtain data that demonstrates he or she is indeed competent and experienced enough to perform it now. Remember: Physicians are not entitled to privileges.

Medical staff leaders should take a hard look at the low-volume providers currently affiliated with the hospital. Are they carrying out patient care activities in the facility at all? Do they only refer their patients to the hospital? Or do they simply seek medical staff membership to maintain a managed care contract?

Develop an 'intended practice plan'

As previously noted, hospitals could include an "intended practice plan" or similar questionnaire with the reappointment packet as a means of determining a physician's level of commitment to the organization. The development of an intended practice plan should be part of the governing body and medical staff's overall strategic planning process. The governing body should carefully review all components of such a plan and adopt it as its official policy. It should certainly consider the recommendations of physician leaders, but, for antitrust or other legal reasons, such recommendations should not be automatically adopted.

If a physician's answers on the questionnaire don't line up with the hospital's criteria for continued membership and privileges, the medical staff office should cease to process the reapplication. Such a move would not constitute a denial of membership, and therefore would not require a report to the National Practitioner Data Bank (NPDB) because they did not meet the criteria for continuation of membership/privileges.

See Figure 7.1 on p. 170 for a sample intended practice plan.

Establish a 'community active' category

If a community-based physician performs little or no work in the hospital, but still demonstrates a strong commitment to the institution (i.e., by referring patients to the hospital) he or she could be reappointed under a "community active" staff category.

The community active category would allow the low-volume physician to refer patients, attend meetings, hold medical staff office, order tests on an outpatient basis, etc., but not hold clinical privileges.

Note: The governing board must approve such a staff category before the hospital may implement it.

See Figure 7.2 on p. 172 for a sample description of the active community-based category.

Establish minimum privileging criteria

The appropriate department chair should write up a report on what he or she deems as the minimum activity level a physician must maintain to competently perform a given procedure. The credentials committee can use this report as a guide when drafting criteria. Remember, JCAHO standards **MS.5.4–MS.5.4.3** require each clinical department to develop its own criteria, "for determining an applicant's ability to provide patient care services within the scope of clinical privileges requested." See Figure 4.3 for a sample worksheet that may be used to develop criteria for specific clinical privileges.

Again, the board must approve all minimum privileging criteria. Once approved, the medical staff should write them into the medical staff bylaws/policies.

Note: It is important to apply minimum privileging criteria equitably to all physicians who request a given clinical privilege. Too often, medical staffs get bogged down with figuring out how to privilege a particular *individual*. But criteria and policies are meant to take the guesswork out of privileging, as they should apply to everyone equally.

If a low-volume provider does not meet the hospital's minimum criteria for a particular privilege, the medical staff office should cease to process his or her privilege request. Again, this move would not constitute a privilege denial and therefore would not warrant a report to the NPDB.

Collect quality and outcomes data

Even with minimum criteria for membership and privileges in hand, how does the medical staff office gather the necessary quality data to determine whether a low-volume provider meets those criteria? The following are some suggestions:

- If a physician is active at another institution, obtain references from the chief executive officer, applicable department chair, and medical records director of that facility. Rather than ask for the traditional reference letters, send a questionnaire that's customized to the individual who will receive it. (See a sample questionnaire for a department chair and a medical records director in Figures 3.31 and 3.33 on pp. 87 and 89.)
- Call the other institution to confirm whether the physician's medical staff status is in good standing with no disciplinary actions, no contemplated investigations, and no ongoing investigations or adverse quality findings. Be sure to document the discussion.
- Inform the physician that it is his or her responsibility to gather the following information from his or her primary hospital:
    - The volume of clinical activity at the facility
    - Confirmation of medical staff status "in good standing" with no disciplinary actions, no contemplated investigations, and no ongoing investigations
    - confirmation from the relevant department chair that the physician is clinically competent in all areas covered by his or her requested privileges
- If a physician is not clinically active at another institution but is active within the community (e.g., a family physician, dermatologist, allergist, etc.), obtain three letters of recommendation from colleagues who are familiar with his or her clinical abilities because they refer patients to, receive referrals from, or otherwise are knowledgeable of his or her ongoing performance.

• Follow up on any incomplete or inadequate information on the questionnaires with a telephone call. If you do not receive the necessary information within the prescribed time frame, cease to process the reapplication. Do not grant clinical privileges.

Physicians who are clinically inactive in any hospital probably aren't qualified to exercise any significant inpatient clinical privileges unless they have recently engaged in substantial continuing medical education or in-hospital training. Because they would not be eligible for significant inpatient privileges, the information needed to verify their competence would be minimal. Turn to Chapter 9 for information on "retraining" physicians who have been out of practice for an extended period of time.

Figure 7.1 | **Sample intended practice plan**

This application contains

- intended practice plan for medical center
- application form
- reference request forms and envelopes

Intended practice plan:

I understand that part of the application process requires me to complete an intended practice plan. I understand that this plan will be used by the health system in developing the conditions for my appointment to the medical staff. I also understand that this plan is not a guarantee or promise that I will actually assist the system in its patient care mission. If I do not assist in any way, I realize that no disciplinary action will be taken and that my appointment will simply expire on the designated date. I also recognize that I have the option of reapplying to the system as an initial applicant if my appointment does, in fact, expire and my practice plans change.

1. I will be establishing or entering practice in one of the areas (specify: _____) designated as an area of need by the system.

If you will not be establishing or entering such a practice, please describe below how you will assist the system in improving patient access to needed services.

_____

_____

_____

_____

2. I expect to assist the system in fulfilling its mission by
   - admitting my patients in need of acute care services to the system for required hospital care
   - scheduling and performing surgery within the system
   - referring patients to the system for definitive consultation, work-up, and management

---

Figure 7.1

Sample intended practice plan (cont.)

If you will not perform or refer patients within the system, how will you assist the system in its patient care mission?

_____

_____

_____

_____

Within your intended practice plan, please address the following issues:

1. I will/will not participate in the hospital's continuing medical education programs to maintain my knowledge and skills. (If not, please describe how you will participate in continuing medical education.)

2. I am/am not employed by a direct competitor of the system (i.e., a hospital or related corporation located within _____ miles of the system). If so, I recognize that I will be ineligible for appointment to the active category of the medical staff.

3. I do/do not own a significant interest in a surgicenter, diagnostic facility, or other inpatient facility that competes directly with patients within the primary or secondary service area of the system. If so, I understand I will be ineligible for appointment to the active category of the medical staff.

4. I absolutely will/will not assist the system in its obligation to provide emergency service to patients in need. (If not, please describe how you plan to assist the health care system in meeting its obligation for emergency patient care.)

5. I will/will not be available to serve on medical staff or hospital committees, task forces, clinical guide-lines development committees, or other medical or administrative committees. (If not, please describe how you assist the system in its medico-administrative activities.)

6. I have/have not arranged for continuing coverage of my patients in the event I am unavailable or unreachable. (If so, please provide a letter signed by the individual or group that has agreed to provide coverage for you. If not, please describe how you will arrange to provide continuous care to your patients if you are unavailable for follow-up, orders, or patient treatment.)

Figure 7.2 **The active community-based category**

All referring category physicians approved by the board as of [insert date] automatically become members of the active community-based category.

Qualifications

Appointees to this category shall consist of medical staff appointees who do not request hospital privileges but want to actively participate in recognized functions of staff appointment, including participation in quality assessment and other monitoring functions, as may be required form time to time. Appointees will do the following:

1. Direct patients to the hospital only through referrals to other members of the medical staff with appropriate privileges for evaluation/admission

2. Complete the application process, but become exempt from medical staff requirements of professional liability coverage

Prerogatives

Appointees may do the following:

1. Visit patients, review medical records, and discuss patient care with the attending physician. No admitting, consulting or surgical privileges are granted.

2. Perform and dictate the preoperative history and physical exams into the hospital record.

3. Order tests and procedures on an outpatient basis.

4. Attend medical staff and department meetings and continuing education meetings.

5. Vote, hold office, and sit on or be the chair of any committee unless otherwise specified in the bylaws.

6. Be afforded the rights of due process.

Figure 7.2 | **The active community-based category (cont.)**

Note: Appointees may not, however, write orders, progress notes, participate in surgery, or actively participate in the direct provision of patient care.

Responsibilities

Appointees shall do the following:

1. Be cognizant of the needs of the hospital. If his or her patient is admitted, he or she must respond in a timely fashion regarding requests for pertinent information on history, medications, allergies, etc.

2. Pay all dues and assessments promptly.

3. Complete the standardized credentialing process for membership.

4. Notify the medical staff office in writing within 30 days of a staff status change at any hospital where membership is held.

5. Participate in the quality review, accreditation, and regulatory compliance requirements for office-based practice as determined by the board.

Chapter 8

Leave

of

Absence

Leave of Absence

Medical staff bylaws generally allow a medical staff member to obtain, for good cause, a voluntary leave of absence (LOA). However, a physician's LOA that exceeds the maximum time limit specified in the medical staff bylaws constitutes a voluntary resignation of medical staff membership and clinical privileges (unless the governing board makes an exception).

Since an LOA results in suspension of the medical staff member's clinical privileges and responsibilities, he or she must formally request termination of the leave as well as the reinstatement of his or her membership status and privileges.

Physicians request LOAs for both personal and business reasons: overseas military assignments, extended education, health issues, and occasionally to avoid a suspension. Medical executive committees (MECs) rarely refuse an LOA request, but it does happen on occasion.

The physician requesting the leave should state the reason motivating his or her request (e.g., to attend an education program, participate in military maneuvers, etc.) and how long the leave will last.

The medical staff bylaws should specify how many days prior to the date the physician wishes to resume practicing at the hospital that he or she must submit the reinstatement request. This enables the hospital to verify the professional activity in which the physician engaged during his or her LOA. If the leave was not for an extended period of time—less than three months—the practitioner should prepare a summary of activities in which he or she participated during the leave. These activities must relate the physician's practice, and he or she must indicate any changes to the information contained in his or her last reappointment application.

If a practitioner's appointment expired during the leave of absence, he or she must complete the full reappointment application.

Letters used to acknowledge and verify relevant information can be adapted from those included in Chapter 3.

Requesting leave

Although a physician's requests for an LOA are rarely contended, hospitals occasionally make more out of such requests than necessary. Remember, there are no laws or accreditation standards that require the MEC to act on LOA requests or the governing board to review such requests for final approval.

Medical staffs may implement a policy that permits the vice president of medical affairs (VPMA), chief of staff, or chief executive officer to review and approve an LOA request under extenuating circumstances, such as when a practitioner leaves for active military duty. A review of such requests by the MEC or governing board would be of little value.

Your credentialing policy should require practitioners to request an LOA in writing, state the reason for the leave, and indicate the estimated start and end dates. Bylaws should outline the procedure to follow when the practitioner returns from leave.

All leave of absence requests should be made in writing to the president of the medical staff, chief executive officer, or the VPMA. Requests should indicate the beginning and ending dates of the requested leave. In addition

- the MEC must reviews all requests and makes a recommendation
- the chief executive officer must forward recommendation to the governing board for action

Requesting reinstatement

When requesting the conclusion of an LOA, the practitioner must submit a written request to the medical staff office for reinstatement with clinical privileges. This request should summarize his or her professional activities during the leave and provide additional information as requested by the hospital.

If the leave was for medical or health reasons, the practitioner must submit a report from his or her attending physician that indicates the physician physically and mentally capable of resuming hospital practice and performing the requested clinical privileges.

Although it is preferable that the hospital receive notice and information in advance of a practitioner's return, it is not always practical, especially when the leave involves military service. Practitioners often forget to send in a request for return 30–60 days in advance (as many bylaws require). Be sure your policies allow practitioners returning from an easily verifiable tour of duty to simply provide a summary of activities and be considered for "return" by the chief medical officer, applicable department chair, and chief executive officer or his or her designee in a timely manner.

Once again, it is not necessary for the MEC or board to consider the request for return unless the situation is unusual or complex (i.e., LOAs taken to avoid a suspension or investigation).

LOAs that extend beyond the physician's regular appointment period are slightly more complex. Under these circumstances, the board can extend the practitioner's appointment until the physician returns. When the practitioner returns, the hospital can immediately process his or her full reappointment following the reappointment process outlined in the hospital's documents. Alternatively, the hospital's policies may dictate that although membership and privileges have lapsed, those membership and privileges can be restored using the reappointment process rather than the more complicated initial appointment process.

The main challenge that hospitals must address upon a practitioner's return from an LOA is the verification of his or her qualifications and current clinical competence. This step requires confirmation of all required credentials and review of the practitioner's activities during the leave. Often the greatest dilemma pertains to the physician's potential skill loss during the leave. Medical staff leaders should assess this issue using common sense and existing hospital policies.

Physicians who return to the hospital after taking an LOA to avoid a suspension or investigation are the most difficult to process. In such situations, the MEC must determine whether the issues prompting the LOA have been resolved. A physician should be permitted to return from leave and practice independently unless the MEC is convinced that such a move would not compromise patient care or the operation of the hospital.

In short, your policies and procedures should make it easy for physicians to request an LOA and return from an LOA. Design documents that allow the hospital flexibility when necessary to avoid making the process overly bureaucratic.

Figure 8.1

Sample bylaws language regarding leaves of absence

Note: The following is a sample excerpt of medical staff bylaws regarding leaves of absence.

The medical staff bylaws define the procedure for leave of absence from [hospital name] to be as follows:

- The board may, for good cause, grant persons appointed to the medical staff a leave of absence for a definitely stated period of time not to exceed one year. Absence for longer than one year shall constitute voluntary resignation of medical staff appointment and clinical privileges unless the board makes an exception.

- Requests for leaves of absence shall be made in writing to the president of the medical staff and to the chief executive officer (CEO), and shall state the beginning and ending dates of the requested leave. The CEO shall transmit the request to the MEC, which shall make a report and a recommendation and transmit it to the CEO for action by the board.

- At the conclusion of the leave of absence, the individual may be reinstated upon filing a written statement with the CEO for transmittal to the MEC summarizing his or her professional activities during the leave of absence. The individual shall also provide other information that may be requested by the hospital at that time.

- If the leave was taken for medical reasons, the individual must submit a report from his or her attending physician indicating that the medical staff appointee is physically/mentally capable of resuming a hospital practice and performing the clinical privileges requested for reinstatement. The individual shall also provide other information that may be requested by the hospital at that time.

- After considering all relevant information, the MEC shall then make a recommendation to the board for final action.

- In acting upon the request for reinstatement, the board may approve reinstatement either to the same or a different staff category, and may recommend limitation or modification of the clinical privileges to be extended to the individual upon reinstatement.

Figure 8.2 — Request for leave of absence

Instructions to the applicant:

Please complete this form to notify *[hospital name]* of your intent to take a leave of absence from the medical staff. Please complete and sign the form and return it to the medical staff office. During the leave, all of your clinical privileges, membership prerogatives, and obligations are suspended. The board may grant a leave of absence for a maximum period of two years. Longer absences will require a new application to the medical staff for appointment and clinical privileges.

Please contact the medical staff office to initiate the process for membership reinstatement at least 60 days before you intend to resume your professional activity at the hospital.

Please type all information.

Name: _____

Assigned department/section: _____

Staff category: _____

Request leave of absence from: ____/____/____ to ____/____/____

Reason for requesting leave: _____

Signature: _____ Date: _____

FOR HOSPITAL USE ONLY

❏ Leave of absence granted for the period indicated above
❏ Leave denied

Reason: _____

Signature: _____ Date:_____

Chair, board of *[trustees]*, *[hospital name]*

| Figure 8.3 | **Leave of absence policy** |

Leave status

A member of the medical staff may obtain a voluntary leave of absence by submitting written notice to the chief of staff, for transmittal to the appropriate department chair and the chief executive officer. The notice must state the approximate time period of the leave, which may not exceed two years, except for military service. During the time period of the leave, the medical staff member's clinical privileges, prerogatives, and responsibilities are suspended.

Termination of leave

The medical staff member must, at least 60 days prior to termination of a leave, or at any earlier time, request reinstatement by sending written notice to the medical staff office for the executive committee's consideration. The medical staff member must submit a written summary of relevant activities during the leave if the MEC or governing board so requests. The MEC makes a recommendation to the governing board concerning reinstatement.

Figure 8.4 Requesting updated information for reinstatement

[Date]

Dear *[Practitioner's name]:*

Thank you for your request to resume your membership and clinical privileges at *[hospital name].*

Step 1: Because your leave of absence exceeded two years or because your appointment to the medical staff expired during your leave or absence or is about to expire, you must reapply for membership and clinical privileges. The necessary forms to initiate this process are enclosed.

Step 2: As part of the reinstatement process, you are required to complete the enclosed *request for reinstatement* form and *request for clinical privileges* form. A copy of your privileges that were in effect prior to your leave is enclosed for your reference.

Please return these documents to the medical staff office, along with a copy of any of the following, which expired during the period of your leave:

- Current license to practice in *[state]*
- Current *[state]*, if applicable, and federal controlled substance registrations
- Face sheet of current professional liability insurance policy, or certificate of insurance, showing coverage limits, expiration, and any exclusions

These materials must be received at least *[30]* days prior to the date on which you anticipate resuming practice at this hospital. Copies of the current medical staff bylaws, rules, and regulations are enclosed. Please read these documents carefully before completing and returning the documents requested.

Sincerely,

[Manager, credentialing services]

Enclosures

Chapter 9

Physician

Retraining

Physician Retraining

When medical staff members return to practice after an extended leave of absence—e.g., to raise a family, to start their own business, to go on sabbatical, to serve in the military overseas, etc.— their clinical skills are often rusty, especially if their leave didn't involve any kind of clinical practice. Such scenarios present a special challenge to credentials committees and medical executive committees (MEC) when faced with reappointing these physicians.

Although a physician may not be completely incompetent to resume practicing medicine (and therefore doesn't warrant a membership and privileges denial), the hospital may feel it's prudent to renew his or her privileges with the condition that he or she works under the supervision of another physician for a prescribed period of time. The hospital may also require the physician to undergo a retraining program to sharpen his or her skills. Once the hospital reviews the physician's progress and deems him or her ready, he or she may resume practicing without supervision.

Use these resources for retraining their medical staff members:

- On-site proctoring/supervision
- Independent training companies

On-site proctoring/supervision

Many hospitals opt to have a returning physician work for an assigned period of time under the direct supervision of a proctor. But who should do the proctoring, who pays for it, and where do proctors come from?

When the department chair, credentials committee, or MEC deems proctoring necessary, it is perfectly appropriate for a competing physician at the hospital to assist with the proctoring. After all, direct competitors are often in the best position to provide information about the quality of the physician's work. Do not, however, require proctors to make recommendations to medical staff leadership or the governing board based on his or her observations. Leave recommendations to the department chair or MEC.

If the medical staff does not have the expertise to proctor a practitioner performing a new procedure, the MEC has the following options:

- Require the practitioner to obtain an appropriately qualified proctor. The hospital will need to perform due diligence to qualify the individual to proctor.
- Assign someone with closely related skills and knowledge to proctor the physician. If necessary, consult an off-site specialist via telephone if a question arises.
- Rather than proctoring, have a team of trained and educated physicians perform procedures along with the practitioner in training. For example, if a cardiologist wants to perform stent placements, appoint an interventional radiologist and a vascular surgeon to the team to ensure that the new procedure goes smoothly.

Compensating proctors is another question altogether. The institution must determine whether a proposed procedure is so critical that it will compensate the proctor. If one physician on staff is authorized to perform a procedure, and the proctored physician wants to perform that procedure outside of the hospital, then that physician could bear the cost of proctoring. The institution is not obligated to compensate the proctor.

Independent training companies

Some companies specialize in retraining medical personnel. Perhaps one of the better-known training companies in the United States today is the Center for Personalized Education for Physicians (CPEP) in Aurora, CO.

The organization, founded in 1990, provides physicians with personalized medical education based on individual educational needs. Unlike traditional continuing medical education (CME), CPEP uses skills and knowledge assessments to identify a physician's weaknesses and develops a customized educational plan to correct those deficiencies.

For many hospitals, access to the resources for conducting an evaluation of a physician's skills presents insurmountable challenges. However, CPEP has access to health care experts and physicians representing a broad spectrum of specialties. An executive director, two assistant directors, a part-time medical director who oversees the clinical aspects of the organization's education and assessment processes, and four administrators staff CPEP.

In addition, the organization contracts with physicians—referred to as associate medical directors—who oversee the assessment and education programs. A pool of approximately 200 board-certified physicians are contracted to conduct a portion of the assessment testing.

CPEP enrollment and assessment

Physicians must submit enrollment information that details the physician's clinical background four to six weeks prior to arriving at CPEP. Although all CPEP assessments evaluate four core areas—knowledge, judgment, documentation, and communication—the background and introductory information gathered during this enrollment phase allows CPEP to develop an individualized assessment program for each physician.

The physician then comes to CPEP to complete a two-day assessment that focuses on the needs identified in the first phase of the process. The assessment includes the following testing components:

Clinical interviews

A physician consultant assigned to the physician conducts clinical interviews during the assessment process. The CPEP associate medical director is also present. The interview is based on charts submitted by the physician, hypothetical case scenarios, and the consultant's case materials. The interview allows the associate medical director to assess the physician's medical knowledge, clinical decision-making process, and documentation practices.

Multiple-choice testing

Multiple-choice tests are customized according to the physician's specialty. (*Note:* CPEP is currently in the process of moving these tests into electronic format.)

Simulated patient encounters

During simulations, actors portray the patients who the physicians would typically treat in their practice. For example, an obstetrician may be presented with an ectopic pregnancy case.

These encounters are videotaped and evaluated by one of three communications experts contracted by CPEP. The communication expert reviews the video and helps the physician understand how he or she can improve communication skills and praises the physician's strengths.

The physicians also document encounters so CPEP consultants can evaluate their "real time" documentation practices. They give the physicians an opportunity to dictate or handwrite their notes, depending on what they are most comfortable with.

Neuropsychological testing

All physicians participating in CPEP's assessment program are required to take a computerized neuropsychological screen. This screen aims to identify signs of early neuropsychological decline. If the test reveals concerns about the physician's performance, further testing is recommended. This testing would occur outside of CPEP.

Specialty-specific testing

The CPEP designs specialty-specific tests that reflect evidence-based medicine and established clinical guidelines. For example, an obstetrician may be asked to interpret fetal-monitoring strips, and a cardiologist may be asked to review electrocardiograms and provide a management plan. The physician's treatment plan is evaluated in accordance with clinical guidelines issued by the relevant specialty association.

Note: It is acknowledged by CPEP representatives that controversy exists across all specialties in regard to some practice guidelines. In cases where a physician's treatment plan differs from a consultant's preferred practice, the consultant determines whether the practice still meets an acceptable standard of care. For example, a clinical guideline for upper respiratory infection may identify the need for a first line antibiotic, but the physician instead may prescribe a secondary drug also identified by the guideline. The drug may not be the ideal, but it could still be acceptable, which is noted.

CPEP evaluates the results of the assessment and issues a final report within four to six weeks. The physician is given an opportunity to review and comment on the report; however, CPEP does not alter its interpretation of the assessment findings. Physicians are permitted to suggest corrections regarding facts such as address, education, background, etc. CPEP gives the physician 10 days to review and sign the report before it distributes the information to the organization that referred the physician (e.g., hospital, licensing board, malpractice insurance carrier).

The assessment determines where on the learning curve each physician's need for education falls. CPEP can then develop educational intervention based on the needs identified by the assessment. This education takes place in the physician's community. CPEP maintains contact with physicians and their education preceptors to monitor activities and progress.

CPEP associate medical directors also conduct ongoing chart review to double-check the preceptor's work to give clinical feedback and direction. In addition, CPEP prepares quarterly reports on the physician's progress, which are sent to the physician and to any referring organizations for review. Once the education is complete, the physician returns to CPEP for a post-education evaluation to ensure that all deficiencies identified by the initial assessment have been corrected.

CPEP retraining

CPEP has discovered that physicians who seek its services because they have been out of the medical field for some time often do very well on the assessment portion of the process because there are often no previous competency concerns in their practice history.

The reentry physicians typically have solid knowledge, decision-making communication, and documentation skills. Any gaps they have can be attributed to their absence from practice and inability to keep up with technology or pharmacotherapeutics

It is difficult for these physicians to go straight into clinical practice at the conclusion of the assessment. Therefore, CPEP has developed an education program that gives the physicians an opportunity to retrain with the assistance and supervision of an experienced peer.

CPEP attempts to organize a retraining program in a university or community hospital setting in the physician's location. The retraining program ensures a smooth transition into clinical practice by incorporating a few months of supervised practice, followed by monitored independent practice lasting between four and six months, depending on the physician's specialty and needs.

CPEP has been able to penetrate some hospitals and university systems that are willing to allow this experience to take place in their facilities with CPEP's oversight, structure, and supervision. However, because this is an emerging trend, establishing such relationships present continuing availability and logistics challenges.

For more information about CPEP, including the cost of assessment and education programs, go to *www.cpepdoc.org*.

State training programs

Many state medical associations and societies have established their own practitioner training programs. While most of these programs were established primarily to assist disruptive or dysfunctional physicians, many also offer retraining for physicians who've simply been out of practice and need to sharpen their clinical skills.

Hospitals contact the Federation of State Physician Health Programs, Inc. (FSPHP) for assistance in finding an appropriate training program within their state. FSPHP is a non-profit corporation that lends support to state programs. The organization provides a forum for the education and exchange of information among state programs to develop common objectives and goals, develop standards to enhance awareness related to physician health and skill, provide advocacy for physicians and their health issues at local, state and national levels, and help state programs protect the public.

To find an FSPHP-affiliated program by state, call 312/464-4574 or go to *www.fsphp.org* and click on "State Program Listing." All states are listed alphabetically in the left-hand column. Click on the desired state for contact information and details about each state program.

Figure 9.1 | # Sample guidelines for proctoring

Note: If your hospital has a different proctoring process in place, replace it with the process that follows below.

I. What is proctoring?

Proctoring is a requirement for medical staff appointment. New members are appointed to the provisional staff upon presentation of adequate and appropriate credentials. Provisional practitioner advancement to the active or courtesy staff category only occurs upon completion of the prescribed proctoring period. Members of the active, affiliate, and courtesy staff who apply for new and additional privileges are also subject to proctoring as defined in these guidelines. Each department needs to individualize its proctoring program.

II. Purpose of proctoring

The purpose of proctoring is to ensure that provisional practitioners are competent in areas of requested privileges. Proctoring is an important part of the privileging process, because it involves both direct observation and assessment of the new staff member's clinical ability. The process of proctoring should assure the proctor, the department chair, the medical executive committee, and the governing body that the new provisional practitioner provides quality care. A well-established system of proctoring is the medical staff's safeguard to prevent compromising quality patient care.

III. Proctoring policy

A. Provisional practitioners shall undergo proctoring for a *[12-month period]*. Under exceptional circumstances, the credentials committee, upon recommendation of the department chair, may extend the period of proctoring. Proctoring begins when the provisional practitioner commences patient care activities.

B. The proctor shall perform proctoring responsibilities by direct observation, as well as by concurrent and retrospective review of the provisional practitioner's cases. The extent of review is determined by the department chair and should be consistent with the breadth of privileges requested. Proctoring reports must be sufficiently detailed to provide an accurate measure of general and specific competency in all categories of privileges requested.

Figure 9.1

Sample guidelines for proctoring (cont.)

C. There shall be a minimum of two proctors for each new staff member.

D. In the reports proctoring reports should include the following:

1. List each case proctored by the patient identification number, type of case, or procedure.

2. Submit each case within 24 hours of the observation.

3. Include the proctor's judgment about the appropriateness of care rendered.

4. Base judgment on direct observation of performance. Retrospective evaluation may be used as a supplement to direct observation. It is recognized that direct observation of psychotherapy and other psychiatric treatments is not possible in all instances; however, direct observation of performance is always desirable.

5. Base judgment on concurrent review until the proctor determines that retrospective review is adequate.

6. Involve all aspects of patient management.

7. Make yourself available to the provisional practitioner.

8. If judgment adverse, forward immediately to the chief of staff/department chair for appropriate action.

9. Include comments regarding the provisional practitioner's ability to diagnose and clinically manage patients, ability to work cooperatively with colleagues, appropriate use of consultants and engender patient confidence.

E. Proctors should not receive a fee for proctoring services. Each proctor should possess sufficient expertise to judge the quality of clinical work performed. In situations where no staff member possesses the qualifications to proctor a provisional practitioner, an outside proctor may be retained by the hospital. Proctors must not be involved in a partnership or financial arrangement with the physician being observed.

Figure 9.1 | # Sample guidelines for proctoring (cont.)

F. The observer/proctor shall not act as an assistant on surgical cases.

G. Evidence of proctoring from a nearby or affiliated institution may be accepted to supplement on-premises observation if the proctor is a member of both medical staffs, is eligible to serve as a proctor in both hospitals and if the same range and level of privileges have been requested by the provisional practitioner in both hospitals.

H. Exceptions to this policy may be made in specific cases only upon recommendation of the credentials committee to the medical executive committee.

IV. Responsibilities of involved parties

A. The department chair shall do the following:

   1. Be responsible for arranging proctoring in accordance with this policy

   2. Appoint the proctors and require them to submit quarterly reports of proctoring activity

   3. Review and endorse the quarterly report and forward it to the credentials committee

   4. Forward a recommendation regarding whether the provisional practitioner should advance to active/courtesy medical staff status at the completion of the proctoring period

B. The credentials committee shall do the following:

   1. Review credentials and other pertinent data supplied by the applicant for privileges and make a recommendation to the board for provisional membership

   2. Review applications for advancement and verify that meaningful proctoring activity has taken place

   3. Review applications for additional proctoring and make a suitable recommendation to the board

---

Figure 9.1 | **Sample guidelines for proctoring (cont.)**

V. Proctoring for additional privileges

A. Members of the active, courtesy, or consulting staff who desire additional privileges shall be proctored for such privileges.

B. The department chair shall determine the extent and scope of proctoring. A specific plan for proctoring shall accompany the application for additional privileges to include the name(s) of the proctor(s) and length of time/number and type of cases to be proctored.

| Figure 9.2 | Sample observation/proctoring program |

Each new medical staff member shall be observed for the following minimum time frames:

Department of family medicine
- First *[5]* admissions to the hospital

Department of surgery
- First *[5]* surgeries

Department of obstetrics and gynecology
- First *[5]* surgeries
- First *[5]* deliveries

Department of pediatrics
- First *[5]* pediatric admissions to the hospital
- First *[5]* newborn admissions to the hospital

Department of medicine
- First *[5]* admissions to the hospital
- First *[5]* electrocardiographic tracings
- Temporary pacemaker insertion; pulmonary artery catheter insertions and management
- Stress test interpretation and monitoring (first *[5]* cases)
- Echocardiogram (first *[5]* cases)
- Gastrointestinal endoscopy (1 case of each of the following)
    - colonoscopy/sigmoidoscopy
    - polypectomy
    - endoscopic retrograde cholangiopancreatography (therapeutic/diagnostic)
- Bronchoscopy (*[5]* cases)
- Renal biopsy (*[1]* case)
- Electroencephalogram interpretation (first *[2]* cases)
- Peritoneal dialysis (first *[2]* cases)
- Diagnostic cardiac catheterization, left heart (*[10]* cases)
- Transesophageal echocardiography (*[10]* cases)

Anesthesia department
- First *[5]* cases
- First delivery and first *[6]* Cesarean sections

Emergency department
- Emergency department medical director evaluates new physicians for a mix of cognitive and procedural skills (*[2]* months)

Pathologists and radiologists
- Over-read of *[5]* slides or films
- Direct observation of invasive procedures (*[10]* mixed cases)

Note: The numbers given above are examples only. Each hospital must determine for itself which time frames make the most sense for the institution.

Figure 9.3 — **Sample proctor assignment procedure**

Procedure

1. The medical staff office, under direction of the relevant department chair, will assign proctors per rotation of qualified members in the relevant specialty.

2. The medical staff office shall do the following:

   • Send a letter to the provisional practitioner and enclose copies of the appropriate department proctoring/evaluation forms. Label each form "I," "2," etc. Provide a #10 envelope stamped "Confidential" that's addressed to the medical staff office. Label the envelopes "I," "2," etc. and staple to the appropriately numbered evaluation form. Instruct the new medical staff member of his or her responsibility to attach the form, with patient name and medical record number, on the medical record and to notify his or her proctor.

   • Send a letter and proctoring protocol to the assigned proctor (and alternate), advising him or her to complete the evaluation form (including the patient name and medical record number), place it in the attached envelope, and seal and return it to the medical staff office.

      Note: If the evaluation form is left on the chart—complete or incomplete—and the medical record is due to be returned to the medical records department, the nurse or medical records clerk will be advised to enclose the form in the envelope and return it to the medical staff office.

   • If the proctor does not complete the form, immediately call the provisional practitioner and advise him or her to ask the proctor to review the chart retrospectively.

   • Request that the chart be pulled and made available to the proctor either in medical records or in the medical staff office.

   • When proctors have been assigned and provisional practitioner(s) notified, the medical staff office will assist in physician compliance by performing the following functions:

      - Review daily report on admissions by admitting/attending physician supplied by the medical records/information services department.

| Figure 9.3 | **Sample proctor assignment procedure (cont.)** |

- Compare the report with the listing of provisional practitioners (i.e., medical staff roster). If any provisional practitioner's name appears on the admit list, call his or her office and remind him or her to contact the proctor (give name of proctor and phone number of office) immediately. Remind him or her of his or her responsibility to attach the proctor form(s) to the medical record so that the proctor can complete the form when he or she evaluates the chart. Once the proctor completes the form, he or she should return it to the medical staff office in the envelope provided.

• As proctor evaluation forms are returned, date stamp and pull the provisional practitioner's credentials file, update the status sheet, and file proctor forms under status sheet. If the case requirement has been met, pull the proctor evaluation forms and status sheet from the file and submit them to the appropriate department chair for review and recommendation.

3. The department chair makes a written recommendation to the credentials committee to advance a practitioner from provisional status, extend the provisional status for a limited period of time, or summarily suspend/terminate the practitioner's privilege(s). The credentials committee makes a recommendation to the medical executive committee to advance a practitioner from provisional status, extend the provisional period for a limited time, or summarily suspend or terminate the practitioner's privilege(s).

Goal: Proctors should complete their proctoring requirements as quickly as possible so provisional practitioners are eligible for advancement from provisional status versus termination of membership/privileges.

Figure 9.4	Letter to appointee regarding medical proctoring procedures

Dear Dr. *[Appointee]*,

On behalf of the department of medicine, I wish to welcome you to *[Hospital name]*. As you know, a proctor will be assigned to observe the care you provide to patients for your first 10 admissions and procedures. Keep a list of these cases and the physician who proctored your work for each.

The purpose of this process is to satisfy the department's obligation to assure the medical community that you are proficient in your specialty and in the delivery of patient care services. Discuss the care plans with the proctoring physician before or upon a patient's admission, at intervals throughout the patient's length of stay/course of treatment, and at discharge.

If I can be of any assistance during your practice here at *[Hospital name]*, please feel free to call me at *[phone number]*.

Sincerely,

[Chair, department of medicine]

Figure 9.5

Letter to appointee regarding surgical proctoring procedures

Dear Dr. *[Appointee]*:

On behalf of the department of surgery, it is my pleasure to welcome you to *[Hospital name]*. As you know, a proctor will be assigned to observe your surgical case and operative proficiency for the first 10 procedures you perform during the first six months of your practice. Keep a list of these cases and note the physician who proctored your work for each.

The purpose of this process is to satisfy the department's obligation to assure the medical community that you are proficient in your specialty and in the delivery of patient care. Discuss each case with the proctoring surgeon—including the preoperative indications and evaluation—before the actual procedure. In addition to intraoperative care, the proctor should evaluate your preoperative and postoperative care.

The operating room is instructed to require the presence of a proctor. It is not their obligation, however, to find a proctor for you. Secure one ahead of time, giving adequate notice to the proctoring surgeon.

If I can be of any assistance during your practice here at *[Hospital name]*, please feel free to call me at *[phone number]*.

Sincerely,

[Chair, department of surgery]

Enclosures

Figure 9.6   **Medical proctor's report**

Patient medical record number: _____

Proctoring physician: _____

Attending physician: _____

Admission date: _____

Discharge date: _____

Setting: _____

Inpatient: _____

Clinic Visit:: _____

Emergency: _____

Other: _____

Diagnosis(es) or chief complaint: _____

Procedure, if relevant: _____

Diagnostic workup (Please use not applicable *[N/A]* when appropriate.)

1. Necessity of admission
   ❏ Appropriate   ❏ Inappropriate*
   Comment: _____

2. Initial level of care/placement
   ❏ Appropriate   ❏ Inappropriate*
   Comment: _____

3. History (promptness, thoroughness, significant negatives, problem-oriented, other)
   ❏ Appropriate   ❏ Inappropriate*
   Comment: _____

4. Physical examination
   ❏ Appropriate   ❏ Inappropriate*
   Comment: _____

5. Problem formulation (initial impression[s], rule-outs, assessment, thoroughness, justification, etc.)
   ❏ Appropriate   ❏ Inappropriate*
   Comment: _____

6. Laboratory use (test selection, sequencing, cost-effectiveness, etc.)
   ❏ Appropriate   ❏ Inappropriate*
   Comment: _____

Figure 9.6 — Medical proctor's report (cont.)

7. Use of diagnostic x-ray/other test modalities or test selections
   ❑ Appropriate   ❑ Inappropriate*
   Comment: _____

8. Initial orders (activity, diet, vital signs, parenteral fluids, clarity, legibility, etc.)
   ❑ Appropriate   ❑ Inappropriate*
   Comment: _____

9. Diagnostic procedures (especially invasive, such as endoscopy, arthroscopy, imaging, biopsies, catheterizations, etc.)
   ❑ Appropriate   ❑ Inappropriate*
   Comment: _____

10. Other _____

Patient management

1. Antibiotic drug use (prophylactic, therapeutic, choice of drug, dosage, route, duration, combinations, toxicity monitoring, serum levels, etc.)
   ❑ Appropriate   ❑ Inappropriate*
   Comment: _____

2. Other drugs (digitalis, glycosides, diuretics, psychotrophics, corticosteriods, anticoagulants, etc.)
   ❑ Appropriate   ❑ Inappropriate*
   Comment: _____

3. Use of blood and blood products
   ❑ Appropriate   ❑ Inappropriate*
   Comment: _____

4. Use of ancillary services (physical therapy, respiratory therapy, social service, dietary, etc.)
   ❑ Appropriate   ❑ Inappropriate*
   Comment: _____

5. Monitoring patient's condition (vital signs, weights, intake/output, follow-up lab tests and x-rays, etc.)
   ❑ Appropriate   ❑ Inappropriate*
   Comment: _____

6. Diet (include parenteral alimentation)
   ❑ Appropriate   ❑ Inappropriate*
   Comment: _____

| Figure 9.6 | **Medical proctor's report (cont.)** |

7. Level of care (include placement, such as intensive care unit, cardiac care unit, stepdown, etc.), activity level, use of isolation, etc.

❏ Appropriate ❏ Inappropriate*

Comment: _____

8. Length of stay

❏ Appropriate ❏ Inappropriate*

Comment: _____

9. Progress notes

❏ Appropriate ❏ Inappropriate*

Comment: _____

10. Complications (anticipated, recognized promptly, dealt with appropriately, etc.)

❏ Appropriate ❏ Inappropriate*

Comment: _____

11. Other: _____

Disposition

1. Placement (transfer, home, extended care facility, home health, etc.)

❏ Appropriate ❏ Inappropriate*

Comment: _____

2. Patient education/instruction (regarding diet, medications, follow-up, level of activity, etc.)

❏ Appropriate ❏ Inappropriate*

Comment: _____

3. Discharge/transfer summary (timeliness, completeness, clarity, legibility, etc.)

❏ Appropriate ❏ Inappropriate*

Comment: _____

Generic competencies

1. Basic medical knowledge

❏ Satisfactory ❏ Unsatisfactory*

2. Clinical judgment

❏ Satisfactory ❏ Unsatisfactory*

Figure 9.6

Medical proctor's report (cont.)

3. Procedural skills
    ❏ Satisfactory   ❏ Unsatisfactory*

4. Communication skills
    ❏ Satisfactory   ❏ Unsatisfactory*

5. Use of consultants
    ❏ Satisfactory   ❏ Unsatisfactory*

6. Professional attitude
    ❏ Satisfactory   ❏ Unsatisfactory*

7. Record-keeping
    ❏ Satisfactory   ❏ Unsatisfactory*

8. Relationship to patient
    ❏ Satisfactory   ❏ Unsatisfactory*

9. Cost-effectiveness
    ❏ Satisfactory   ❏ Unsatisfactory*

Please explain below or on the reverse side.

General comments on the handling of this case: _____
_____
_____

Proctoring physician's signature: _____ Date _____

Note: Thank you very much for your assistance in reviewing this physician. Your comments are of great value to the medical executive committee. Once you have completed this form, please return it to the chair of the department of medicine.

Please do not photocopy or share this confidential report with anyone except the attending physician or the department chair.

Figure 9.7

Surgical proctor's report

Part I and II (to be completed at the time of surgery)

Patient medical record number: _____

Proctoring surgeon: _____

Primary surgeon: _____

Date & time: _____

Chief complaint: _____

Surgical procedure(s): _____

Emergency case   ❏ Yes   ❏ No

Preoperative

1. H&P on chart and complete   ❏ Yes   ❏ No
2. Progress note(s) regarding planned procedure complete   ❏ Yes   ❏ No
3. Preoperative justification for surgery documented   ❏ Yes   ❏ No

General comments: _____

_____

_____

Intraoperative

Please comment on the following, if applicable: Punctuality of primary surgeon; technical skill; knowledge of procedure; blood loss; surgical judgment; conduct in operating room; etc. *Continue on a separate sheet if necessary.*

Comments: _____

_____

_____

Note: Thank you very much for your assistance in reviewing this surgeon. Your comments are of great value to the surgical committee. Once you have completed this form, please return it to the surgical department chair.

Proctoring surgeon's signature: _____ Date _____

Please do not photocopy or share this confidential report with anyone except the attending physician or the surgical department chair.

Figure 9.8

Surgical proctor's report—Part III

Part III (to be completed when this information becomes available)

Patient medical record number: _____
Proctoring surgeon: _____
Primary surgeon: _____
Date & time: _____
Chief complaint: _____
Surgical procedure(s): _____

Postoperative

1. Does preoperative diagnosis coincide with postoperative findings?   ❏ Yes   ❏ No

2. Was postoperative care adequate?   ❏ Yes   ❏ No

3. Was operative report complete, accurate, and timely?   ❏ Yes   ❏ No

4. Were complications (if any) recognized and managed appropriately   ❏ Yes   ❏ No

General comments on the handling of this case: _____
_____
_____
_____

Note: Thank you very much for your assistance in reviewing this surgeon. Your comments are of great value to the surgical committee. Once you have completed this form, please return it to the surgical department chair.

Proctoring surgeon's signature: _____ Date _____

Please do not photocopy or share this confidential report with anyone except the attending physician or the surgical department chair.

Figure 9.9 | **Letter accompanying provisional status report**

Re: *[Appointee name]*
Date: *[Appointment date:]*
Staff category: *[Active, courtesy, etc.]*
Department: *[Insert name]*
Section/specialty: *[Insert name]*

Dear credentials committee chair:

I am pleased to report that the above-named provisional practitioner has demonstrated his or her qualifications for staff appointment and for his or her staff category. He or she has also satisfactorily demonstrated his or her ability to exercise the privileges initially granted.

The findings documented in the attached report are based upon my review of this appointee's credentials file, including a summary of his or her activities during his or her provisional period and observed performance. Therefore, I recommend that his or her provisional status be concluded.

If you have any questions concerning this report or the practitioner's qualifications and clinical competence, please contact me at *[phone number]*.

Sincerely,

[Department chair]
Enclosures

Chapter 10

Avoid

Credentialing and

Reappointment

Mistakes

Avoid Credentialing and Reappointment Mistakes

In reappointment, reappraisal of a physician's clinical competency is critical since that is where most liability risk arises for hospitals. Courts across the country have concluded that hospitals owe a duty to their patients to exercise reasonable care in selecting physicians for their medical staffs and in granting clinical privileges.

Therefore, hospitals can't afford to take reappointment and privileging decisions lightly, or have incomplete/ineffective reappointment policies and procedures in place.

Review: Two types of failures

As noted in Chapter 1, mistakes in initial appointment occur because of to two types of failures. The first is *mechanical failure*. Mechanical failure is the inability to collect all relevant information concerning a new applicant to support a membership/privileges decision. Mechanical failure is occasionally due to the absence of policies and procedures requiring the collection of all appropriate information. Under other circumstances, it happens as the result of an organization's inability to obtain information even when it believes such information is necessary for appropriate, well-informed decision-making.

The second type of failure is referred to as *decision failure*, which much more complex. Decision failure occurs when those entrusted with the responsibility of making membership and privileges recommendations do so unwisely. Such decisions could be attributed to competitive issues, blind faith, the need for expediency, or the inappropriate belief that physicians should be given the benefit of the doubt under all circumstances.

An excellent medical staff services professional (MSSP), armed with contemporary credentialing policies, will almost always eliminate the possibility of mechanical failure. It is not difficult today to gather all of the necessary information regarding a physician's background. But if it should become difficult, shift the burden onto the applicant. See Chapter 1, Figure 1.1 for a sample policy and procedure. All processing should cease until the applicant provides complete, accurate, and verifiable information about his or her past.

The elimination of decision failure comes only with a focused sense of purpose, personal integrity, and experience. When complex credentialing issues arise, there is no substitute for a seasoned credentials committee composed of five to seven individuals who are highly trained, well-educated, and dedicated to the medical staff process.

Credentialing root-cause analysis

Another way to prevent future reappointment mistakes is to conduct a root-cause analysis (RCA) when a major failure is identified. Many industries, such as the nuclear power industry, commercial airlines, and the United States military use RCAs to investigate "sentinel events" to determine their cause(s) so policies and procedures can be changed as appropriate. A "sentinel event" is defined as any unexpected clinical or nonclinical occurrence that results in loss of life or bodily harm, disrupts operations, or threatens the organization's assets and reputation. This definition also includes "near misses," or any breakdown in process that carries the risk of a serious adverse outcome.

Credentials committees might benefit significantly from conducting a careful RCA whenever a failure or near miss occurs in the credentialing process. The following credentialing-related sentinel events are worthy of an RCA:

1. Any fair hearing, termination, or denial of medical staff appointment or clinical privileges
2. A corporate negligence suit alleging improper or inadequate credentialing
3. A nasty privileging turf battle
4. Any time it takes more than 100 days to process a medical staff application/reapplication or a clinical privileges request

Each of the above scenarios might be considered a sentinel event, thereby prompting the formation of an RCA team composed of individuals familiar with such analyses.

Conducting an RCA

The first step involved in conducting an RCA is to assign a team to assess the sentinel event. Such teams may need to be established on an ad hoc basis, or the core of an appropriate team may already exist in the form of a targeted performance improvement– or some other team. The team should include staff at all levels closest to the issue involved, those with decision-making authority, and individuals critical to the implementation of potential recommended changes.

Note: It's not necessary for all team members to be thoroughly experienced in credentialing; it's more important to have members who are willing to ask "Why?" for the fifth time when attempting to determine the actual cause of a breakdown or near miss.

The team should

- have its core members and leader/facilitator clearly defined
- be empowered to do its assessment and make changes or recommendations for changes
- be provided the resources, including time, to do its work
- have a defined structure and process for moving forward

At the beginning of the process, the team leader or facilitator should establish a way of communicating team progress and findings to senior leadership. Keeping senior leaders informed on a regular basis is critical to management support of the RCA initiative and implementation of its recommendations. Although it is difficult to provide guidelines on what constitutes "on a regular basis," as this will vary widely depending on circumstances.

The creation of a detailed action plan is also critical to the process and to securing management support. A plan outlining target dates for accomplishing specific objectives provides a tool against which to guide and measure the team's progress. The full work plan should include target dates for major milestones and key activities in the root cause analysis process, including

- defining the event and identifying the proximate and underlying causes
- collecting and assessing data about proximate and underlying causes
- designing and implementing interim changes
- identifying the root causes
- planning improvement
- testing, implementing, and measuring the success improvements

Figure 10.1 is a tool for organizing the steps in an RCA.

Note: Not all possibilities and questions listed will apply in every case, and others may emerge during the course of analysis.

Criminal background checks

Still another way to avoid credentialing failures—and to protect patient safety and the organization's reputation—is to conduct criminal background checks on all medical staff applicants. Some hospitals feel such a step is unnecessary because state medical boards already check physicians' backgrounds before they issue licenses. In reality, very few boards conduct such checks.

Criminal background investigations are not new to some areas of health care. For example, many states require organizations to conduct criminal background investigations on home health care workers since these people are going into patients' homes. In California, the state Respiratory Care Board requires respiratory therapists to submit fingerprints with their applications, which the board then runs through federal and state background investigations for criminal convictions.

In addition, Illinois enacted legislation in August 1997 that requires criminal background investigations on all workers who have direct patient contact. Also in 1997, all new medical license applicants in Florida had to submit their fingerprints to the Florida Board of Medicine. And in 2000, all physicians in Florida had to submit their fingerprints for license renewal.

Conducing criminal background investigations on employees but not physicians presents a double standard that is difficult to defend in court. Also, to complicate the issue further, what about those physicians who are employed by the hospital?

Where to find information

As of yet, there are no industry standards or consensus on what crimes to look for when checking an individual's criminal history, or how far into the person's past to delve. Hospitals may want to check for all crimes—both federal and state, felonies and misdemeanors. Some of the available resources for researching criminal background are as follows:

- **County court records.** These require a lot of time as they require a visit to each courthouse in person. The hospital must determine all places in which the practitioner lived, worked, or attended school going back a reasonable period of time. The best way to verify that the physician has listed all previous locations on an application is to run a check on the Social Security number through a screening or credit company. It is reasonable to search the past 10 years, and if it raises red flags, hospitals can always search further back. Note: Most courts only keep records for seven to 10 years.
- **FBI database.** This is the only national database accessible to health care organizations that contains information about federal, state, and local crimes. However, not all states and localities report to it, and there is no penalty if they don't.
- **State databases.** Most states have statewide crime databases, but they are often incomplete. Combine state and county searches for a more complete record.
- **Sex offender registry (SOR).** These registries were originated under Megan's Law, which requires sex offenders to register with law enforcement authorities in the state when they

move to a new locality. Check the SOR in conjunction with county court records. In most states, one can simply go online to check the SOR at *www.ojp.usdog.gov/hjs/abstract/sssor01.htm* or call the Megan's Law Helpline at 631/689-2672.

- **Federal court records.** This type of search also requires an in-person visit the courthouse.

If a hospital does not have the resources to conduct such checks through its medical staff office, it could consider using a screening company or asking the human resources department to help. Most hospitals already have processes in place to conduct checks on nonphysician employees.

Tips for developing a system

If a hospital decides that conducting criminal background checks is important, but is worried about the cost, there are ways to develop an effective investigation system to help keep expenses down. Consider the following recommendations:

- Know your state law. Criminal investigations must be done in accordance with state law to avoid invasion of privacy concerns. Inform applicants that you will conduct criminal background investigations.
- Determine how you are going to treat cases that were settled without a finding.
- Consider making the criminal investigation the final element of an employee's probation or a physician's privileges. When employees are hired, they can be advised that you will perform a criminal investigation and will use that information to determine whether they will keep their job. All other aspects of their performance can be assessed before spending the money on the criminal investigation.
- Develop and follow your policy. It is important to determine how far back you are willing to look into an employee's or a physician's criminal background. Also, apply the policy without discrimination.
- Contract with an employee screening company. That company can do the work for you more thoroughly, completely, and efficiently.

The bottom line: By taking extra measures—such as criminal background checks—to ensure that the quality and competence of their physicians, hospitals will avoid credentialing and privileging mistakes, thereby protecting patient safety, guarding against negligent credentialing litigation, and making the reappointment process much easier.

Figure 10.1	Guide to the credentialing root-cause analysis process

Preparation for the root-cause analysis

Step I: Identify the event or condition to be analyzed (i.e., which step in the credentialing process appeared to fail?)

Step II: Gather, verify, and store information (e.g., credentials files and work forms)

Step III: Assign a team leader and team facilitator to lead the analysis team

Step IV: Conduct analysis

Step V: Engage in decision-making

First analysis team meeting

- Introduce team members
- Establish expectations
- Identify ground rules
- Describe the methodology
- Designate a "Parking Lot"
- Identify the proximate (or immediately obvious) cause(s) of the event
- Generate a detailed sequence of events with pertinent process flowcharts
- Brainstorm to identify potentially contributory factors
- Edit and correlate all the brainstorm items
- Set the date and time for the next meeting

Between the first and second analysis team meetings

- Determine whether the error was due to a poor process or decision failure
- Process failure involves a lack of information (e.g., licensure, malpractice coverage, education, training, disciplinary actions, etc., not verified properly)
- Decision failure involves leaders not considering all pertinent information or failing to act in a timely manner
- Assign other team members to collect any data identified as necessary

---

Figure 10.1

Guide to the credentialing root-cause analysis process (cont.)

Second analysis team meeting

- Present contributory factor diagram to the team
- Finalize the contributory factor diagram, identifying root causes or root contributors
  Note: *The actual root-cause analysis is now complete. The action plan and report must now be generated.*

Between the second and third analysis team meetings

- Prepare several copies of the contributory factor diagram for distribution to the team
- Complete as much as possible of the root cause analysis report form, and prepare several copies for distribution to the team

Third analysis team meeting (occasionally requires two meetings)

- Present contributory factor diagram for final approval to the team
- Generate at least one corrective or improvement action for each identified root cause or root contributor
- Address "Parking Lot" items
- Establish plan for communication of analysis report.

Final report

1. Team leader and facilitator finalize written report
2. Submit report to local risk management advisory committee for approval
   - If approved
     - terminate team
     - distribute report
   - If not approved
     - use shortfalls identified by advisory committee to guide root-cause analysis team in remediation
     - resubmit report for approval
     - distribute report

Chapter 11

Practical

Tips

Practical tips

This chapter contains practical tips for tackling challenges that arise during reappointment, between appointment and reappointment, or while of doing business. These tips come from hospital administrators, medical staff services professionals, and The Greeley Company consultants.

Evaluate your credentialing and recredentialing policies

Near the end of each calendar year—around November or December—your credentials committee and medical staff office should take stock of its credentialing and recredentialing policies and procedures. It should identify strengths and weaknesses by reviewing and analyzing the hospital's current processes.

Follow the below suggested guidelines.

1. **Develop and distribute questionnaires.**
Distribute a questionnaire to medical staff leaders that allows them to evaluate the effectiveness of the hospital's credentialing and recredentialing program. Send a second questionnaire to all medical staff members to solicit feedback about the program as well as to provide physicians with information on how the credentialing and reappointment processes work.

2. **Compile an annual report**
The annual report should include the following information:

- A subjective appraisal of the credentialing and recredentialing program as generated by the above-mentioned questionnaires
- The number of initial applicants processed in the past year
- The number of reapplicants processed in the past year
- The number of resignations and retirements processed in the past year
- The average time span between receipt of an (re)application and board approval

- The number of instances in which temporary privileges were granted, the reason for granting the temporary privileges, and time necessary to process these requests
- The number of instances between appointment and reappointment where there were changes in staff category (e.g., from active to courtesy or courtesy to active)
- The number of instances between appointment and reappointment in which additional or modification of privileges were requested
- Any instances in which a turf battle arose, and the amount of time spent handling these complex issues
- The number and duration of credentials committee meetings
- The overall costs associated with the credentialing program
- An evaluation of the credentials verification organization (if applicable)

Once you have gathered all of the above information, the credentials committee chair, the VPMA/manager of medical staff services, and the chief of staff should perform a preliminary analysis of the data, identify performance improvement targets, identify problem areas, and develop a plan for process improvement. The plan should then be submitted to the credentials committee and MEC for consideration. These committees should review and discuss the identified problems, and recommend new procedures, policies, or systems to improve the viability and effectiveness of the programs.

There are great benefits to conducting a year-end analysis of these programs. The credentials committees and medical staff offices should conduct such an analysis within the next 12 months.

You could start by using the sample self-assessment tool, which can be found in Figure 11.1 on page 229, to design your own evaluation process.

Conduct exit and post-appointment interviews

Medical staff leaders, hospital leaders, and the MEC could benefit from adopting a common business practice used in other industries: the exit interview.

Over the course of a year, medical staffs are faced with physician retirements, voluntary resignations, and relocations. These departing physicians often possess information that could help the MEC and hospital administration improve its operations.

Exit interviews allow hospitals to gather departing physicians' impressions about the hospital, and its benefits structure, management style, and interpersonal relations.

The medical staff leadership should review and evaluate the results of exit interviews. Hospital administration would also benefit from a review of the interview findings.

Several hospitals across the country have modified the standard exit interview to use with new medical staff members. They use it to obtain the new member's assessment of the organization's application process, orientation structure, and availability of information about the hospital. These interviews are frequently called post-appointment interviews, and are often conducted by a current medical staff member.

The post-appointment interview may also provide the hospital with valuable information about the appointment and orientation practices of competing hospitals.

Exit and post-appointment interviews should be straightforward, and conducted by a neutral party who is skilled in asking questions and documenting answers. For example, an employee from human resources or public relations department would be a fine choice.

Remember, the objective of exit interviews and post-appointment interviews is to gather data that can guide the modification of cumbersome, bureaucratic, or unnecessary practices that the hospital casually adopted over time.

Late return of reappointment applications

Tardy reapplication materials are one of the most common reappointment obstacles faced by the medical staff office. The failure of physicians to submit all necessary documentation results in large number of unprocessed reappointments requests.

To remedy this situation, hospitals may opt to send a letter to the physician informing him or her that the time period within which the practitioner was to submit an application for reappointment and clinical privileges has ended. The hospital may inform the physician that failure to submit the reappointment application is an indication of his or her wish to voluntarily relinquish appointment and privileges. However, the organization should allow the physician request that his or her reappointment file be reopened in accordance with medical staff bylaws.

Many hospitals have attempted to remedy this situation by levying late fines and allowing the appointment to expire. Keep in mind, however, that tardy reapplications are the medical staff office's problem only if it assumes they are. This problem rightly belongs to the chief of staff or VPMA. Inform the MEC president of which physicians are too busy, too fed up with bureaucracy, or too forgetful to return their reapplications on time. The MEC president should then communicate this information to the chief of staff or VPMA.

A call from the chief of staff to a tardy physician most often results in the prompt return of needed reappointment paperwork.

In the meantime, the medical staff office should concentrate on processing the reapplications of those physicians who follow the organization's reappointment polices and procedures.

Find answers to your NPDB questions

The National Practitioner Data Bank's (NPDB's) most recently updated guidebook (published in September 2001) is now available free of charge on its Web site. This guide, an invaluable resource for medical staff offices and credentials committees, explains events that are reportable to the data bank, and tells which health care entities must submit such reports.

To access the guidebook, go to *www.npdb-hipdb.com/guidebook.html* and click on "Guidebooks" under the "Publications" heading in the left-hand column. You can download the guide in its entirety or by section.

See also Appendix D for a sample NPDB policy.

Waive dues and reapplication fees

Consider waiving medical staff dues and reapplication fees for physician leaders who give many volunteer hours to the medical staff. This is an incentive for physicians to serve the medical staff, and provides a small recognition of existing leaders' dedication and service. The decision to waive such fees does not require a bylaws change. The MEC must simply reach an agreement on the issue. Inform the rest of the staff that this reward is for those physicians who give their time and energy to the medical staff.

Credentialing processes and insurance rates

Could your credentialing processes be a liability risk? As the malpractice insurance crisis continues to capture the attention of health care executives and physicians, your credentialing procedures may fall under the scrutiny of insurance providers.

Your hospital may strive to implement effective credentialing programs to satisfy state, federal, and accreditor standards and to ensure the competency of your medical staff. But as your organization grapples with the realities of the malpractice insurance crisis, it may find yet another reason for revamping weak credentialing and recredentialing policies and procedures—the potential for reduced liability insurance rates. Some insurers offer discount rates for organizations that demonstrate solid credentialing practices.

Medical Assurance Inc., based in Birmingham, AL, is one of several insurance companies that now offers "sizable" insurance discounts for complying with criteria that focus on high risk-areas, including credentialing and clinical outcomes data.

Credentialing is one component of Medical Assurance's risk mapping surveys which are conducted at each of its insured facilities four or five times a year. Risk mapping surveys began almost 20 years ago when the company first started insuring hospitals.

The insurer began to focus on credentialing due to the number of allegations filed against its insureds that called into question the competency of physicians and other hospital staff.

Although many of the details Medical Assurance looks for in credentialing files coincide with various accreditors' requirements, its requirements are based solely on issues that have been difficult for them to defend in past lawsuits.

During the risk mapping survey, Medical Assurance's surveyors meet with the hospital's medical staff coordinator for approximately 30 minutes to determine whether the organization

- appropriately credentials and recredentials medical staff members
- provides physicians with continuing medical education
- maintains quality improvement/peer review information on medical staff members
- queries the NPDB
- has a mechanism to identify a change in privileges
- has a mechanism to verify competency of physicians who perform privileges outside their normal scope of practice

Surveyors review several credentialing files during the risk-mapping survey to determine whether the organization meets the insurer's requirements (specified previously). The surveyors typically review credentials files for

- an obstetrician performing an epidural (if applicable)
- a newly appointed physician
- a newly reappointed physician
- a certified registered nurse anesthetist
- a gastroenterologist administering conscious sedation
- a nurse practitioner with privileges

- a nurse midwife with privileges,
- a physician-employed nurse involved in patient care or who makes rounds with/for a physician
- a physician-employed surgical assistant

Surveyors also review medical staff bylaws that address continuing medical education requirements and privileges, and allied health protocols.

Note: Compliance with each set of criteria is scored on a scale of one to four. For example, a Medical Assurance surveyor would review a newly appointed physician's file to determine whether medical staff members are appropriately credentialed. The surveyor would check whether the file contained an application, current licensure information, specific training and clinical experience information, peer recommendations regarding clinical competency, professional liability actions, voluntary or involuntary relinquishment of licensure, voluntary or involuntary loss of membership or privileges, and consent for inspection of records. An organization receives a score of four if all required information is in the file.

If the insurer detects areas that need improvement, it suggests remedies to the organization. Medical Assurance then monitors the organization's progress—if the organization decides to respond to the suggestions—during return visits.

Medical Assurance sends the findings of the risk mapping surveys to its underwriting department, which then determines whether an organization qualifies for a discount. The discount is based on whether the organization's policies and procedures are satisfactory, whether areas of needed improvement are detected, and whether the organization has acted on previous recommendations.

External peer review

Does your hospital have a policy clearly describing the circumstances under which it would seek the assistance of an external peer review organization? If not, you might want to put one in place before your next JCAHO survey.

JCAHO standards MS.8-MS.8.4 require a hospital to define situations in which it will seek external peer review. These definitions must be incorporated into the medical staff policies.

There are six general situations that often require external peer review: litigation, ambiguity, lack of internal expertise, conflict of interest, new technology, and miscellaneous issues. (Be sure to specify these situations in your policy.)

- **Litigation**—Hospital legal counsel often contact external peer review organizations when the hospital faces a potential medical malpractice suit. External peer review organizations are called on to provide an expert opinion regarding quality of care.

- **Ambiguity**—Confusion can arise when groups conducting an internal review reach conflicting conclusions that will affect a practitioner's membership or privileges. When internal reviewers submit conflicting or vague recommendations, or fail to reach a common understanding, the situation can often be resolved by turning to an external organization to review the applicable records.

- **Lack of internal expertise**—Many hospitals, particularly rural facilities, are occasionally forced to rely on external peer review organizations because medical staff members do not have expertise in the specialty under review. External peer review organizations are also called in when the only practitioners on the medical staff with expertise to review the specialty are associates, partners, or direct competitors of the practitioner under review.

Note: Your medical staff policy regarding external peer review may specify that external organizations will be used if potential conflicts of interests can not be appropriately resolved by the MEC or governing board.

- **New technology**—Hospitals that acquire new technology may discover they do not have the necessary tools to assess whether a medical staff member requesting privileges associated with the new technology possesses the required skills and competence. See Chapter 4 on clinical privileging and how to develop criteria for special procedures, including new technology.

- **Miscellaneous issues**—Most hospitals adopt external peer review policies that allow the MEC and governing board to use external peer review whenever deemed appropriate (e.g., when the medical staff needs an expert witness for a fair hearing, to evaluate a practitioner's credentials file, or to develop benchmarks for quality monitoring.)

Note: If your hospital must rely on external review, it is important that you find a credible resource to provide that service. Make certain that the external peer review organization will still be in business in two years to provide fair hearing testimony if necessary.

In addition, the organization should have a large physician consultant panel, a longstanding track record, reviewers who are board certified in the specialty that needs reviewing, and reviewers who actively participate in health care improvement are detected, and whether the organization has acted on previous recommendations.

The importance of due diligence

The Associated Press recently reported that a surgeon in Hawaii chose to implant the shaft of a screwdriver into a patient's spine when he could not locate the proper titanium stabilization device. If proven true, this story suggests a terrible lapse of judgment on the part of the surgeon, but would not necessarily indicate a problem with the hospital's credentialing process. Hospitals cannot be expected to be clairvoyant and anticipate such isolated incidents.

However, the hospital must immediately improve its processes if it knew of problems in the physician's past and failed to consider them, or if it failed to conduct thorough primary-source verification.

What could the hospital in Hawaii have discovered about the physician's past that may have alerted it to potential performance problems? The above incident occurred on January 29, 2001. According to the results of a background check conducted through the Fraud Abuse Control Information Service (FACIS), operated by Government Management Services, Inc. (*www.facis.com*), the Oklahoma State Board of Medical Licensure and Supervision suspended the physician's license and issued a five-year probation in January 1999.

If the hospital had conducted a background check, it would have also discovered that the Texas State Board of Medical Examiners revoked the physician's license in April 2000, and that the physician was included on the Office of Inspector General's list of excluded practitioners in 1994 and 1996. However, timing may not have allowed the hospital to uncover information about the negative action taken by the Kansas State Medical Board of Healing Arts in 2002.

Clearly, due diligence would have disclosed this surgeon's questionable past. One can only wonder what action a diligent credentials committee would recommend when faced with an application from a physician with such a record.

Figure 11.1	**Credentialing self-assessment**

Initial appointment process

1. Do you have written policies and procedures for the initial appointment process? ☐ Yes ☐ No

2. Does the governing body approve all credentialing policies and procedures? ☐ Yes ☐ No

3. Do current medical staff bylaws, board bylaws, or a separate document describe the roles, responsibilities, functions, relationships, and authorities of the following:
   - Governing board? ☐ Yes ☐ No
   - Chief executive officer? ☐ Yes ☐ No
   - Medical executive committee? ☐ Yes ☐ No
   - Credentials committee? ☐ Yes ☐ No
   - Medical staff? ☐ Yes ☐ No
   - Department chair? ☐ Yes ☐ No

4. Is your credentialing process ongoing? ☐ Yes ☐ No

5. Do you follow the same credentialing procedures for all practitioners? ☐ Yes ☐ No

6. Do you consistently apply credentialing criteria? ☐ Yes ☐ No

7. Are your credentialing criteria objective and rational with respect to the hospital's business and quality-of-care concerns? ☐ Yes ☐ No

8. Do you process applications within the time frame specified in the medical staff bylaws? ☐ Yes ☐ No

9. Does each applicant to the medical staff submit
   - a formal application for appointment? ☐ Yes ☐ No
   - a statement regarding his or her
     - physical and mental health status*? ☐ Yes ☐ No
     - impairment due to chemical dependency/substance abuse? ☐ Yes ☐ No

*All healthcare organizations must comply with the Americans with Disabilities Act.

- history of loss of license/felony convictions?	❑ Yes	❑ No
- history of loss or limitation of privileges or disciplinary activity?	❑ Yes	❑ No
• an attestation to the correctness and completeness of his or her application?	❑ Yes	❑ No

10. For each applicant, do you obtain and verify from primary sources

• a current, valid license?	❑ Yes	❑ No
• clinical privileges in good standing?	❑ Yes	❑ No
• a valid Drug Enforcement Administration (DEA) or Controlled Dangerous Substance (CDS) certificate?	❑ Yes	❑ No
• board certification status?	❑ Yes	❑ No
•graduation from medical school and completion of residency, or board certification (if applicable)?	❑ Yes	❑ No
• clinical practice history?	❑ Yes	❑ No
• current professional liability insurance coverage, including coverage for the privileges requested (according to hospital policy)?	❑ Yes	❑ No
• professional liability claims history?	❑ Yes	❑ No

11. Do you request information from the following sources for each applicant:

• The National Practitioner Data Bank (NPDB)?	❑ Yes	❑ No
• The State Board of Medical Examiners or Department of Professional Regulations?	❑ Yes	❑ No
• The American Medical Association (AMA) Physician Masterfile?	❑ Yes	❑ No
• The American Board of Medical Specialties (ABMS)?	❑ Yes	❑ No
• The American Osteopathic Physician Profile?	❑ Yes	❑ No
• The Board Action Data Bank of the Federation of State Medical Boards (FSMB)?	❑ Yes	❑ No
• The Chiropractic Information Network/Board Action Databank (CINBAD), when appropriate?	❑ Yes	❑ No
• The National Register of Health Service Providers in Psychology, if applicable?	❑ Yes	❑ No
• The HHS, Office of the Inspector General (OIG), for a list of excluded individuals and entities?	❑ Yes	❑ No
• Appropriate individuals at the practitioner's previous practice settings/hospital affiliations?	❑ Yes	❑ No

12. Do you have written procedures for

• obtaining any missing or additionally required information from the applicant?	❑ Yes	❑ No

- closing the applicant's file if he or she does not respond to requests for additional information in a timely manner?   ❑ Yes   ❑ No

13. Do you delegate any credentialing activities to a CVO, do you
    - oversee and monitor the CVO's activities?   ❑ Yes   ❑ No
    - maintain written documentation specifying
        - any delegated activities?   ❑ Yes   ❑ No
        - the CVO's accountability for credentialing functions?   ❑ Yes   ❑ No

14. Do you present only completed files to the department chair for review?   ❑ Yes   ❑ No

15. Does the credentials committee review requests for and make recommendations for temporary privileges?   ❑ Yes   ❑ No

16. Does the credentials committee make all recommendations on medical staff appointment and clinical privileges to the MEC?   ❑ Yes   ❑ No

17. Does the MEC make final recommendations to the board concerning credentialing decisions?   ❑ Yes   ❑ No

18. Does your hospital routinely consider the impact of credentialing decisions on
    - the quality of patient care?   ❑ Yes   ❑ No
    - the medical staff"   ❑ Yes   ❑ No
    - the hospital?   ❑ Yes   ❑ No

19. Does your hospital grant medical staff membership only to qualified individuals?   ❑ Yes   ❑ No

20. Do you have a fair hearing plan that gives practitioners the opportunity to appeal adverse credentialing decisions?   ❑ Yes   ❑ No

21. Has your fair hearing plan been recently reviewed by appropriate legal counsel?   ❑ Yes   ❑ No

22. Do you report all adverse decisions (through the state medical board) to the NPDB?   ❑ Yes   ❑ No

23. Do you orient all new appointees to their roles and responsibilities?   ❑ Yes   ❑ No

24. Do you have policies and procedures for monitoring the performance of all new medical state members for a provisional period?   ❏ Yes   ❏ No

Privileging

25. Do you have written policies and procedures for delineating clinical privileges?   ❏ Yes   ❏ No

26. Do the written criteria for granting of privileges include
    - the physician's
        - prior and continuing education and training?   ❏ Yes   ❏ No
        - prior and current experience?   ❏ Yes   ❏ No
        - utilization practice patterns?   ❏ Yes   ❏ No
        - current health status*?   ❏ Yes   ❏ No
        - documented competence and judgment to provide high-quality, appropriate services in an efficient manner?   ❏ Yes   ❏ No
        - geographic location?   ❏ Yes   ❏ No
    - patient-care needs for the type of privileges being requested?   ❏ Yes   ❏ No
    - current/anticipated practice volume?   ❏ Yes   ❏ No
    - the hospital facility's ability to accommodate the requested privilege(s)?   ❏ Yes   ❏ No
    - availability of qualified coverage in the practitioner's absence?   ❏ Yes   ❏ No
    - the level of professional liability insurance the physician must have to perform or provide the requested procedures or treatments?   ❏ Yes   ❏ No

27. Do you query the NPDB
    - for all requests for temporary privileges?   ❏ Yes   ❏ No
    - for initial appointment and reappointment?   ❏ Yes   ❏ No
    - for all requests for additional privileges between initial appointment and reappointment?   ❏ Yes   ❏ No

28. Does your hospital grant clinical privileges only to qualified individuals?   ❏ Yes   ❏ No

Reappointment process

29. Do you have written policies and procedures for the reappointment process?   ❏ Yes   ❏ No

30. Do you review and reverify the credentials of each practitioner at least every two years?   ❏ Yes   ❏ No

31. Do you reverify (with primary sources) at least the following information: ❑ Yes ❑ No
- A current, valid license? ❑ Yes ❑ No
- Clinical privileges in good standing? ❑ Yes ❑ No
- A valid DEA or CDS certificate? ❑ Yes ❑ No
- Board certification (if applicable)? ❑ Yes ❑ No
- Work history? ❑ Yes ❑ No
- Current professional liability insurance and coverage for the privileges granted (according to hospital policy)? ❑ Yes ❑ No
- Professional liability claims history? ❑ Yes ❑ No

32. Do you receive from each practitioner a statement regarding his or her
- physical and mental health status? ❑ Yes ❑ No
- impairment due to chemical dependency or substance abuse? ❑ Yes ❑ No

33. Do you request information from the following sources:
- the NPDB? ❑ Yes ❑ No
- the State Board of Medical Examiners or Department of Professional Regulations? ❑ Yes ❑ No
- the AMA Masterfile? ❑ Yes ❑ No

34. Do you review the following information for each practitioner:
- Physician utilization statistics? ❑ Yes ❑ No
- Continuing medical education? ❑ Yes ❑ No
- Department, general staff, and committee meeting attendance? ❑ Yes ❑ No
- Medical records completion? ❑ Yes ❑ No
- Participation in emergency room on-call schedule? ❑ Yes ❑ No
- Clinical activity statistics? ❑ Yes ❑ No
- Incident reports? ❑ Yes ❑ No
- Reports of disciplinary action? ❑ Yes ❑ No
- Data bank reports, as listed above? ❑ Yes ❑ No

35. Do you complete a reappointment activity summary or profile for each applicant for reappointment? ❑ Yes ❑ No

Disciplinary matters

36. Do you have policies and procedures that address
- impaired physicians? ❑ Yes ❑ No
- sexual harassment? ❑ Yes ❑ No

      • conflict resolution within the medical staff regarding any aspect of
the credentialing/privileging process in dispute?   ❑ Yes   ❑ No

      • leave of absence?   ❑ Yes   ❑ No

      • sharing or exchange of medical staff information?   ❑ Yes   ❑ No

37.   Does your hospital:

      • reduce, suspend, or terminate clinical privileges as necessary?   ❑ Yes   ❑ No

      • report disciplinary actions to appropriate authorities?   ❑ Yes   ❑ No

      • have an appeal process for practitioners who have been
disciplined?   ❑ Yes   ❑ No

      • inform practitioners of the procedure by which they may appeal any
disciplinary action?   ❑ Yes   ❑ No

Documentation

38.   Do you store credentials files in a secure location?   ❑ Yes   ❑ No

39.   Are credentials files easily accessible?   ❑ Yes   ❑ No

40.   Do you have a policy/procedure controlling the confidentiality
of credentials information?   ❑ Yes   ❑ No

41.   Do you have a policy/procedure regarding access to and
release of credentials information?   ❑ Yes   ❑ No

42.   Do you maintain updated information regarding

      • physician utilization statistics?   ❑ Yes   ❑ No

      • continuing medical education?   ❑ Yes   ❑ No

      • department, general staff, and committee meeting attendance?   ❑ Yes   ❑ No

      • medical records completion?   ❑ Yes   ❑ No

      • participation in emergency room on-call schedule?   ❑ Yes   ❑ No

      • clinical activity statistics?   ❑ Yes   ❑ No

      • incident reports?   ❑ Yes   ❑ No

      • reports of disciplinary action(s)?   ❑ Yes   ❑ No

      • data bank reports?   ❑ Yes   ❑ No

Appendix

Figure A

Sample initial appointment policy

The hospital will forward all requests for applications to the medical staff to the medical staff office. After the medical staff office receives an application request, it will send an application package with a cover letter to the potential applicant. The letter should state that the hospital will accept and process applications for only those applicants who can demonstrate that they can fulfill the following:

- Have completed (or are in the last six months of) an approved residency program of at least three years' duration
- Have actively practiced at least six of the last 12 months (residency included), have actively practiced in an accredited hospital at least two of the past five years, or have two years of recent experience in a full-time clinical residency
- Have established, or plan to establish, an office and residence within 30 minutes of this hospital, unless the applicant is joining a group and at least one half of that group lives within the specified distance, or can provide other acceptable evidence of patient coverage
- Are currently licensed to practice in this state
- Maintain professional liability insurance in an amount specified by the board
- Are board-certified or board-admissible

The application package shall include the following:

- An application for appointment to the medical staff
- A privileges delineation overview
- Privileges request forms and criteria for privileges
- A detailed list of requirements for completing the application

In addition, the medical staff office shall provide (or make available) to the applicant a copy of the medical staff bylaws overview or a complete set of medical staff bylaws, rules, and regulations.

If the application meets the preapplication criteria stated in the application package cover letter, the hospital will accept the application. The medical staff office will initiate a credentials file for each individual requesting medical staff membership or clinical privileges.

The application must be typed and on the form designated by the credentials committee and approved by the board.

Conditions of appointment

In signing the application, the applicant

Figure A

Sample initial appointment policy (cont).

- attests to the accuracy and completeness of all information on the application and any accompanying documents and agrees that any inaccuracy, omission, or commission is grounds for terminating the application process
- signifies his or her willingness to appear for interviews regarding his or her application, peer review, and hospital quality improvement activities
- authorizes hospital and medical staff representatives to consult with prior and current associates and with others who might have information bearing on his or her professional competence, character, ability to perform the privileges requested, ethical qualifications, ability to work cooperatively with others, and other qualifications for membership and the clinical privileges he or she requests
- consents to hospital and medical staff representatives' inspection of all records and documents that might be material to an evaluation of his or her professional qualifications and competence to carry out the clinical privileges requested, physical and mental health status[1], and professional and ethical qualifications
- releases from liability—to the fullest extent permitted by law—any and all hospital representatives for acts they perform and statements they make in connection with evaluation of his or her application, credentials, and qualifications
- releases from liability all individuals and organizations who provide information to the hospital or the medical staff, including release to hospital representatives of otherwise privileged or confidential information concerning the applicant's background, experience, competence, professional ethics, character, physical and mental health[1], emotional stability, utilization practice patterns, and other qualifications for staff appointment and clinical privileges
- authorizes and consents to hospital representatives providing other hospitals, medical associations, licensing boards, and other organizations concerned with practitioner performance and the quality and efficiency of patient care, with any information relevant to such matters that the hospital may have concerning him or her, and releases hospital representatives from liability for so doing
- signifies that he or she has read the current medical staff bylaws and associated manuals and agrees to abide by their provisions in regard to his or her application for appointment to the medical staff
- agrees to provide to the medical staff office updated information requested on the original application and subsequent reapplications or privilege request forms, including the following:

  - Hospital appointments
  - Voluntary or involuntary relinquishment of medical staff membership or clinical privileges, or licensure status
  - Voluntary or involuntary limitation
  - Reduction or loss of clinical privileges at another hospital
  - Involvement in liability claims, or license/DEA sanctions (including both current and pending investigations and challenges)

Figure A

Sample initial appointment policy (cont).

- Any removal from a managed care organization's provider panel for quality-of-care reasons or unprofessional conduct
- agrees to disclose any successful or currently pending challenges to licensure or registration or voluntary or involuntary relinquishment of such licensure or registration to the medical staff office or chief executive officer (CEO);
- agrees to disclose voluntary or involuntary termination of medical staff membership or voluntary or involuntary limitation, reduction, suspension, or loss of clinical privileges at another institution
- agrees to disclose any current clinical charges pending, and any past charges and convictions of misdemeanors or felonies

For the purposes of this provision, the term "hospital representatives" includes the following entities:

- The board, its directors, and committees
- The CEO or his or her designee
- Registered nurses and other employees of the hospital
- The medical staff organization and all medical staff appointees
- Clinical units and committees that have responsibility for collecting and evaluating the applicant's credentials or acting upon his or her application
- Any authorized representative of any of the aforementioned.

Procedure for processing applicants for initial staff appointment

The applicant must provide the following information necessary to complete the application:

- A typed, completed, and signed application form and request for privileges.
- A copy of current state license and, where applicable, DEA certificate.
- A copy of the face sheet of the current professional liability insurance policy or certificate of insurance.
- Copies of certificates or letters confirming completion of an approved residency/training program or other educational curriculum.
- Copies of certificates or letters from appropriate specialty board(s) stating board status—e.g., board qualification or board certification, or recertification.
- Names and addresses of three professional references who have recently worked with the applicant and has directly observed his or her professional performance over a reasonable period of time. At least one reference must be an individual practicing in a field similar to that of the applicant. (The hospital will directly contact the references and request information regarding current clinical ability, ethical character, and ability to work with others.)

Figure A

Sample initial appointment policy (cont).

If the medical staff office does not receive all of the above information within 45 days of receipt of the application, the hospital will consider the application incomplete and the medical staff office will suspend further processing. The hospital will send one reminder notice to the applicant after the medical office receives the application, noting missing items or information.

After receiving a completed application as defined above, the CEO will send a letter of acknowledgment to the applicant. The medical staff office will then post the applicant's name, specialty, and board status in the designated area to permit current medical staff members to provide additional information regarding the applicant to the credentials committee.

The medical staff office will then verify the application's contents and collect additional information as follows:

- Information from all prior and current insurance carriers concerning claims, suits, and settlements (if any) during the past five years
- Administrative and clinical reference questionnaires from all significant past practice settings for the previous 10 years
- Verified documentation of the applicant's past clinical work experience
- Verification of licensure status in all current or past states of licensure
- Information from the AMA Physician Masterfile or Federation of State Medical Boards
- Verification of completion of medical, osteopathic, dental school and residency, fellowship programs
- Information from the National Practitioner Data Bank.
- Information from the Office of Inspector General relevant to Medicare/Medicaid sanctions, if applicable

Note: If there is undue delay in obtaining required information, the medical staff office will request assistance from the applicant. If the applicant fails to respond adequately to a request for assistance within 30 days of the hospital's request, the hospital will terminate the application process.

When the medical staff office has obtained the above items, it will summarize the file on an Executive Summary form and present the file to the appropriate department chair and the credentials committee chair.

The department chair or credentials committee chair shall make at least one telephone call to solicit additional information from past practice settings. Documentation of this contact will be placed in the credentials file.

Figure A

Sample initial appointment policy (cont).

Clinical interview

Policy

It is this hospital's policy that the department chair, credentials committee chair, or other member of the credentials committee shall conduct a clinical interview for each new applicant for medical staff appointment and/or privileges. The permanent record of the interview shall include the general nature of questions asked, the adequacy of answers, and the conclusion of the committee (group) or interviewer regarding the applicant's qualifications for membership and/or requested privileges.

The interviewer may solicit information to complete the credentials file or clarify previously provided information, such as the applicant's past malpractice history, reasons for leaving past health care organizations, or other matters bearing on the applicant's ability to render high-quality care.

Generally, no applicant will be recommended to the board of directors for appointment or privileges without first participating in a personal interview. An exception will be made in those instances in which officers or credentials committee members already know the candidate. The department chair or credentials committee chair will complete an interview form in any case.

Procedure

The applicant is responsible for contacting the department chair to arrange the interview. The applicant will be notified when the verification process is complete so that he or she can contact the department chair or credentials committee chair to schedule an interview.

If the applicant fails to schedule an interview with the designated medical staff leader, the application will be considered incomplete and no further processing will take place. The applicant will be notified of the incomplete status of the application.

The medical staff leader/committee who conducted the interview must complete an Interview Report and place it in the applicant's credentials file.

Effect of department chair report

After the department chair receives the application from the medical staff office, he or she reviews the application to ensure that it fulfills the established standards for membership and clinical privileges.

Deferral: The department chair may not defer consideration of an application. He or she must forward a report to the credentials committee within 15 days. If, for some reason, the chair is unable to formulate a report, he or she must so inform the credentials committee and the applicant.

Figure A

Sample initial appointment policy (cont).

Favorable recommendation: The department chair must document his or her findings pertaining to adequacy of education, training, and experience for all requested privileges. He or she should document and include in the credentials file any reference to criteria for privilege review. The department chair must then forward his or her recommendation, the application, and all supporting documentation to the credentials committee.

Adverse recommendation: The department chair must document his or her rationale for all unfavorable findings. He or she should document and include in the credentials file all references to any unmet criteria for clinical privileges. The CEO shall promptly notify the applicant of the adverse recommendation by special written notice. The department chair shall then forward his or her adverse recommendation with the application and supporting documentation to the credentials committee.

Effect of credentials committee action

Upon receipt of the department chair's recommendation, the credentials committee reviews the application to ensure that it fulfills the established standards for membership and clinical privileges.

Deferral: If the credentials committee defers the application for further consideration, the committee must make recommendations as to approval or denial of—or any special limitations to—staff appointment, category of staff and prerogatives, department affiliations, and scope of clinical privileges within 30 days. The CEO shall promptly notify the applicant of the action to defer by special written notice.

If the credentials committee's conclusions contradict those of the department chair, the credentials committee and the department chair shall meet to discuss the differences. A written summary of the discussion and conclusions shall be prepared as an addendum to the credentials committee's report.

Favorable recommendation: When the credentials committee's recommendation is favorable to the applicant in all respects, the credentials committee shall promptly forward its recommendation, the application, and all supporting documentation to the medical executive committee (MEC).

Adverse recommendation: When the credentials committee's recommendation is adverse to the applicant, the CEO shall notify the applicant of the adverse recommendation by special written notice. The credentials committee shall forward the application, supporting documentation, and all dissenting views to the MEC.

MEC action

Upon receipt of the credentials committee's recommendation, the chair of the MEC (chief of staff) reviews the application to ensure that it fulfills the established standards for membership and clinical privileges.

Figure A

Sample initial appointment policy (cont).

Deferral: If the MEC defers the application for further consideration, it must recommend approval or denial of—or any special limitations to—staff appointment, category of staff and prerogatives, department affiliations, and scope of clinical privileges within 30 days. The chief of staff shall promptly notify the applicant by special, written notice of the action to defer.

Favorable recommendation: When the MEC's recommendation is favorable to the applicant in all respects, the application shall be forwarded, together with all supporting documentation, to the board.

Adverse recommendation: When the MEC's recommendation is adverse to the applicant, a special notice shall be sent to the applicant. No such adverse recommendation will be forwarded to the board until after the practitioner has exercised or has waived his or her right to a hearing as provided in the medical staff bylaws.

Board action

Upon receipt of the MEC's recommendation, the CEO (or designee)—whom the board has authorized to approve the appointment and clinical privileges on its behalf—reviews the application and all supporting documentation.

Favorable recommendation: The board may adopt or reject—in whole or in part—a favorable recommendation of the MEC or may refer the recommendation back to the MEC for further consideration, stating the reasons for such referral and setting a time limit within which it must make a subsequent recommendation. Favorable action by the board is effective as its final decision.

Adverse recommendation: If, after complying with the requirements, the board's action is adverse to the applicant, a special written notice will be sent to the applicant, and he or she shall be entitled to the procedural rights as stated in the fair hearing provision in the medical staff bylaws.

After the fair hearing: In the case of an adverse MEC recommendation, the board shall take final action in the matter as provided in the medical staff bylaws.

Basis for recommendation and action

Each individual or group that is required to act on an application—including the board—must state the reasons for each recommendation or action taken, with specific reference to the completed application and any other relevant documentation. Any dissenting views at any point in the process must also be documented, supported by reasons and references, and transmitted with the majority report.

Figure A

Sample initial appointment policy (cont).

Conflict resolution

If the board determines that its decision will contradict the MEC's recommendations, it will submit the matter to a committee comprising an equal number of MEC and board members. The committee shall review the information and submit its recommendation to the board within 30 days of the date on which the board submitted the matter.

Notice of final decision

The CEO shall notify the MEC and the chair of each relevant department of the board's decision. The applicant shall receive written notice of appointment and special written notice of any adverse final decisions.

A decision and notice of appointment includes

- the staff category to which the applicant is appointed
- the department to which he or she is assigned
- the clinical privileges he or she may exercise
- any special conditions attached to the appointment or exercise of clinical privileges

Time periods for processing

Individual/group	Time period
• Medical staff office (to collect and summarize)	60 days
• Department chair (to review and recommend)	15 days
• Credentials committee (to reach final recommendation)	30 days
• Medical executive committee (to reach final recommendation)	30 days
• Board of directors (to render final decision)	30 days

All individuals and groups required to act on an application for staff appointment must do so in a timely manner and in good faith. Unless there is good cause, each application should be processed within the following time periods:

The time periods listed above are merely guidelines and do not create any right to have an application processed within these precise periods. If the provisions of the fair hearing plan are activated, the time requirements provided therein govern the continued processing of the application.

Figure B — Impaired or dysfunctional physician policy

Background

The problem of impairment is complex, and the investigation and hearing process is not appropriate in this situation. The American Medical Association (AMA) defines the impaired physician as "one who is unable to practice medicine with reasonable skill and safety to patients because of a physical or mental illness, including deterioration through the aging process or loss of motor skill, or excessive use or abuse of drugs, including alcohol." This policy is intended to provide some overall guidance and direction on how to proceed when confronted with a potentially impaired physician.

Because of the independent nature of most physicians' practices and the serious implications of any disability, an impairment is often difficult to identify early and is always difficult for the impaired physician to acknowledge. It is hard to face the problem with a physician. For all these reasons, the problem often goes unaddressed for too long. Nevertheless, it is the obligation of the hospital and medical staff leadership to address it. The following policy provides the framework within which to do it.

Because the term "impaired physician" includes a variety of problems, from age to substance abuse to physical or mental illness, the steps provided below will not be suitable in every circumstance. There can be no one policy to cover all situations. Specific needs and varying circumstances preclude a single inflexible mechanism for dealing with all impaired physicians. The number and seriousness of incidents involving a physician, for example, may dictate the appropriate response by the hospital. If the "investigation" suggested in the policy is carried out, the individuals conducting the investigation will vary from hospital to hospital, depending upon personalities, circumstances, and the structure of the medical staff. Whichever mechanism a hospital chooses, the risk of patient harm must be of paramount concern. Immediate action may be necessary.

One exception to this policy is impairment due to age and irreversible medical illness or other factors not subject to rehabilitation. In such cases, the sections of the policy dealing with rehabilitation and reinstatement of the physician are not applicable.

Key factors to keep in mind while dealing with any issue relating to a physician's illness or disability are state reporting statutes and the application of the Americans with Disabilities Act. These policies should, under any interpretation of the law, be legally appropriate, as with all matters with significant legal implications. Legal counsel should be consulted.

Note: The chief executive officer (CEO) plays a significant role in this process in conjunction with medical staff leadership. That is because an impaired physician is a hospital concern, not merely a medical staff problem.

Figure B

Impaired or dysfunctional physician policy (cont.)

Report and investigation

If any individual working in the hospital has a reasonable suspicion that a physician appointed to the medical staff is impaired, the following steps should be taken:

1. The individual who suspects the physician of being impaired must give an oral or, preferably, written report to the CEO or the medical staff president (or the physician's help committee). The report must be factual and shall include a description of the incident(s) that led to the belief that the physician might be impaired. The individual making the report does not need to have proof of the impairment, but must state the facts that led to the suspicions.

2. If, after discussing the incident(s) with the individual who filed the report, the CEO or the medical staff president believes there is enough information to warrant an investigation, the CEO shall request that an investigation be conducted and a report of its findings rendered by one of the following:

   (a) The medical staff president

   (b) A standing committee of the medical staff

   (c) An outside consultant

   (d) Another individual or individuals appropriate under the circumstances

3. If the investigation produces sufficient evidence that the physician is impaired, the CEO shall meet personally with that physician or designate another appropriate individual to do so. The physician shall be told that the results of an investigation indicate that the physician suffers from an impairment that affects his or her practice. The physician should not be told who filed the report, and does not need to be told the specific incidents contained in the report.

4. Depending upon the severity of the problem and the nature of the impairment, the hospital has the following options:

   (a) Require the physician to undertake a rehabilitation program as a condition of continued appointment and clinical privileges

   (b) Impose appropriate restrictions on the physician's practice

   (c) Immediately suspend the physician's privileges in the hospital until rehabilitation has been accomplished, if the physician does not agree to discontinue practice voluntarily

Figure B — Impaired or dysfunctional physician policy (cont.)

5. The hospital shall seek the advice of hospital counsel to determine whether any conduct must be reported to law enforcement authorities or other government agencies, and what further steps must be taken.

6. The original report and a description of the actions taken by the CEO or medical staff president should be included in the physician's personnel file. If the investigation reveals that there is no merit to the report, the report shall be destroyed. If the investigation reveals that there may be some merit to the report, but not enough to warrant immediate action, the report shall be included in a confidential portion of the physician's personnel file and the physician's activities and practice shall be monitored until it can be established whether there is an impairment problem.

7. The CEO or medical staff president shall inform the individual who filed the report that follow-up action was taken.

8. Throughout this process, all parties shall avoid speculation, conclusions, gossip, and any discussions of this matter with anyone outside those described in this policy.

9. In the event there is an apparent or actual conflict between this policy and the bylaws, rules, regulations, or other policies of the hospital or its medical staff—including the due process sections of those bylaws and policies—the provisions of this policy shall supersede such bylaws, rules, regulations, or policies.

Rehabilitation

10. Hospital and medical staff leadership shall assist the physician in locating a suitable rehabilitation program. The hospital shall not reinstate a physician until it is established, to the hospital's satisfaction, that the physician has successfully completed a rehabilitation program in which the hospital has confidence.

Reinstatement

11. Upon sufficient proof that a physician who has been found to be suffering an impairment has successfully completed a rehabilitation program, the hospital may consider reinstating that physician to the medical staff.

12. When considering an impaired physician for reinstatement, the hospital and its medical staff leadership must consider patient-care interests to be paramount.

13. The hospital must first obtain a letter from the physician director of the rehabilitation program where the physician was treated. The physician must authorize the release of this information. The letter from the director of the rehabilitation program shall state

Figure B

Impaired or dysfunctional physician policy (cont.)

(a) whether the physician is participating in the program

(b) whether the physician is in compliance with all of the terms of the program

(c) whether the physician attends program meetings regularly (if appropriate)

(d) to what extent the physician's behavior and conduct are monitored

(e) whether, in the opinion of the rehabilitation program physicians, the physician is rehabilitated

(f) whether an aftercare program has been recommended to the physician and, if so, a description of the aftercare program

(g) whether, in the program director's opinion, the physician is capable of resuming medical practice and providing continuous, competent care to patients

14. The physician must inform the hospital of the name and address of his or her primary care physician, and must authorize the physician to provide the hospital with information regarding his or her condition and treatment. The hospital has the right to require an opinion from other physician consultants of its choice.

15. The hospital shall request the primary care physician to provide information regarding the precise nature of the physician's condition, the course of treatment, and the answers to the questions posed above in 13 (e) and (g).

16. Assuming all information the hospital receives indicates that the physician is rehabilitated and capable of resuming patient care, the hospital must take the following additional precautions when restoring clinical privileges:

(A) the physician must identify two physicians who are willing to assume responsibility for the care of his or her patients in the event that he or she is unable or unavailable to care for them

(B) the hospital shall require the physician to provide the hospital with periodic reports from his or her primary care physician—for a period of time specified by the CEO and the medical staff president—stating that the physician is continuing treatment or therapy, as appropriate, and that his or her ability to treat and care for patients in the hospital is not impaired

Figure B

Impaired or dysfunctional physician policy (cont.)

17. The department chair or a physician appointed by the department chair shall monitor the physician's exercise of clinical privileges in the hospital. The credentials committee shall determine the nature of that monitoring after reviewing all of the circumstances.

18. The physician must agree to submit to an alcohol or drug screening test (if appropriate to the impairment) at the request of a member of hospital management, a physician, or a nurse who suspects that the physician may be under the influence of drugs or alcohol.

19. All requests for information concerning the impaired physician shall be forwarded to the CEO for response.

Figure C

Disruptive medical staff members policy

Policy

It is the policy of this hospital that all individuals within its facilities be treated with courtesy, respect, and dignity. To that end, the board requires that all individuals, employees, physicians, and other independent practitioners conduct themselves in a professional and cooperative manner in the hospital or on hospital property.

If an employee fails to conduct himself or herself appropriately, the matter shall be addressed in accordance with human resources policies. If a physician or other independent practitioner fails to conduct himself or herself appropriately, the matter shall be addressed in accordance with the following policy. It is the intention of this hospital that this policy be enforced in a firm, fair, and equitable manner.

The board of trustees will address disruptive behavior by physicians and other independent practitioners. A single egregious incident such as physical or sexual harassment, assault, a felony conviction, a fraudulent act, stealing, damaging hospital property, or inappropriate physical behavior may result in immediate termination of employment or medical staff membership. The board may, at its discretion, refer such issues to the medical executive committee for investigation and recommendation.

Objective

The objective of this policy is to ensure optimum patient care by promoting a safe, cooperative, and professional health care environment, and to prevent or eliminate—to the extent possible—conduct that

- disrupts the operation of the hospital
- affects the ability of others to do their jobs
- creates a "hostile work environment" for hospital employees or other medical staff members
- interferes with an individual's ability to practice competently
- adversely affects or impacts the community's confidence in the hospital's ability to provide quality patient care

Guidelines

A single egregious incident or repeated incidents shall initiate investigative action according to the hospital's policy on appointment. Summary suspension may be appropriate pending this process.

In the event such action is based solely upon disruptive conduct, the practitioner will not be afforded a "fair hearing" as defined in medical staff policies. A single appeal to the board or an appellate committee of the board will be permitted. If it is unclear whether the conduct was actually disruptive, the board may seek the expert opinion of an impartial individual experienced in such matters.

Figure C

Disruptive medical staff members policy (cont.)

Unacceptable disruptive conduct may include, but is not limited to, behavior such as the following:

1. Attacks—verbal or physical—leveled at other appointees to the medical staff, hospital personnel, patients, visitors or others encountered as a result of association with this hospital, that are personal, irrelevant, or beyond the bounds of fair professional conduct

2. Impertinent and inappropriate comments (or illustrations) made in patient medical records or other official documents, impugning the quality of care in the hospital, or attacking particular physicians, nurses, or hospital policies

3. Nonconstructive criticism that is addressed to its recipient in such a way as to intimidate, undermine confidence, belittle, or imply stupidity or incompetence

4. Refusal to accept—or disruptive acceptance of—medical staff assignments or participation in committee or departmental affairs regarding anything but his or her own terms

Documentation of disruptive conduct is critical because it is ordinarily not one incident that leads to disciplinary action, but rather a pattern of inappropriate conduct. Such documentation shall include

- the date and time of the questionable behavior

- a statement of whether the behavior affected or involved a patient in any way, and, if so, the name of the patient

- the circumstances that precipitated the situation

- a description of the questionable behavior that is limited to factual, objective language

- the consequences, if any, of the disruptive behavior as it relates to patient care or hospital operations

- a record of any action taken to remedy the situation, including the date, time, place, action, and name(s) of those intervening

Any physician, employee, patient, or visitor may report potentially disruptive conduct. The report shall be submitted to the medical director or a facility administrator and then forwarded to the chief executive officer, medical director, or the president of the medical staff.

Figure C

Disruptive medical staff members policy (cont.)

Once received, the medical director, in consultation with the president of the medical staff, will investigate the report. The medical director may dismiss unfounded reports. The individual initiating such report will be appraised. Those reports considered accurate will be addressed as follows:

1. A single confirmed incident warrants a discussion with the offending physician; the medical director or designee shall initiate such a discussion and emphasize that such conduct is inappropriate and must cease. The initial approach should be collegial and helpful to the physician and the hospital.

2. If it appears to the medical director and/or the president of the medical staff that a pattern of disruptive behavior is developing, the medical director or designee shall discuss the matter with the physician as outlined below:

   • Emphasize that if such repeated behavior continues, more formal action will be taken to stop it. The MEC and CEO will be notified.

   • All meetings shall be documented.

   • A follow-up letter to the physician shall state the nature of the problem and inform the physician that he or she is required to behave professionally and cooperatively within the hospital.

   • The involved physician may submit a rebuttal to the charge. Such rebuttal will be maintained as a permanent part of the record.

3. If such behavior continues, the CEO, board chair, or designee shall meet with and advise the physician that such conduct is intolerable and must stop. This meeting is not a discussion, but rather constitutes the physician's final warning. It shall be followed with a letter reiterating the warning.

This policy shall be the sole process for dealing with egregious incidents and disruptive behavior, and shall be interpreted and enforced by the board. No other policy or procedure shall be applicable to egregious incidents or disruptive behavior except as designated by the board.

Note: Hospitals must seek expert legal advice when implementing this policy and procedure. Provisions of this recommended policy might conflict with existing medical staff bylaws or fair hearing procedures. Hospitals must address such conflicts before finalizing this policy.

Policy on the National Practitioner Data Bank

Figure D

I. Authorized represpentative

The hospital's authorized representative for sending reports to and receiving queries from the National Practitioner Data Bank shall be the chief executive officer (CEO) or another hospital employee designated in writing by him/her.

II. Queries

A. Queries to the data bank about applicants for medical staff appointment and/or clinical privileges shall be made routinely as part of the initial application verification process. Such queries shall be made prior to transmitting the application to the department chair.

B. Queries on applicants for reappointment shall be made routinely as part of the regular reappointment verification process. Such queries shall be made prior to transmitting the application to the department chairs. The CEO, or designee, shall maintain a record establishing that a query has been made at least every two years for every individual appointed to the medical staff.

C. Appointments, clinical privileges, and reappointments shall be conditional until a response from the data bank is received.

D. Copies of all information obtained through queries to the data bank shall be maintained as part of the individual's permanent confidential medical staff credentials file.

E. The board's credentials committee may at any time request that the CEO make a query to the data bank with respect to any individual appointed to the medical staff. The CEO may also determine to make a query on his/her own.

III. Reports

A. A report shall be made to the data bank (via the state board of medicine) within fifteen (15) days of final board action on any of the following:

1. denial of initial medical staff appointment
2. denial of medical staff reappointment
3. revocation of medical staff appointment
4. denial of initial clinical privileges
5. denial of request for increased clinical privileges
6. decrease of clinical privileges

Figure D

Policy on the National Practitioner Data Bank (cont.)

    7. suspension of clinical privileges for longer than thirty days

    8. imposition of mandatory concurring consultation requirement

B. If an individual resigns his/her medical staff appointment or clinical privileges, the credentials committee shall make a preliminary determination as to whether such resignation constitutes surrender while under investigation or surrender in return for not conducting an investigation. The committee's preliminary determination shall be reported to the CEO by the committee chairperson or his/her designee. A final determination as to whether a report is required shall be made by the CEO after consultation with hospital counsel.

C. For the purpose of reporting a surrender of medical staff appointment or clinical privileges to the data bank, an investigation shall be deemed to have commenced when the credentials committee determine by resolution to initiate an investigation. The credentials committee may pass such a resolution on its own motion, or after receiving a written request for an investigation.

D. The reason(s) for the action taken shall be described on the Adverse Action Report and shall be, to the extent possible, as follows:

    1. clinical competence or judgment below hospital standard

    2. lack of sufficient training and/or experience to demonstrate current clinical competence

    3. violation of hospital or medical staff bylaws, rules and regulations, or policies

    4. violation of condition(s) placed on the exercise of initial, temporary, or locum tenens clinical privileges

    5. conduct that disrupts the orderly operation of the hospital

    6. impairment caused by alcohol abuse

    7. impairment caused by substance abuse

    8. inability to work cooperatively with others

    9. psychiatric impairment

    10. physical impairment

    11. misrepresentation or omission of facts

    12. conviction of a criminal offense

E. The CEO shall determine what language shall be used after consulting with the chairperson of the credentials committee and the chief of staff, and after obtaining the advice of hospital counsel.

Figure D
Policy on the National Practitioner Data Bank (cont.)

IV Resolving Disputes

A. The data bank will provide every individual with a copy of any report made about him/her. The data bank shall also provide a process by which an individual can dispute the factual accuracy of a report that has been filed.

B. The first step in this process is to attempt to resolve any dispute with the hospital. In the event that an individual wishes to dispute the accuracy of an Adverse Action Report submitted by the hospital, the individual shall state in writing to the CEO the reason why he/she believes the report to be factually inaccurate.

C. The CEO shall then consult with the chairperson of the credentials committee, the chief of staff, and hospital counsel. Within 30 days of receipt of the written notice by the individual disputing the accuracy of the Adverse Action Report, the CEO shall notify the affected individual of the hospital's decision whether or not to revise the information previously reported to the data bank.